PocketGuide to Treatment in Speech-Language Pathology

PocketGuide to Treatment in Speech-Language Pathology

M. N. Hegde, Ph.D.
Department of Communicative
Sciences and Disorders
California State University-Fresno

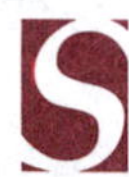

SINGULAR PUBLISHING GROUP, INC.
SAN DIEGO · LONDON

Singular Publishing Group
401 West "A" Street, Suite 325
San Diego, California 92101-7904

e-mail: singpub@singpub.com
web site: http://www.singpub.com

Second Printing May 1996
Third Printing July 1997
Fourth Printing May 1998
Fifth Printing September 1999

Typeset in 9/11 Stemple Schneidler by So Cal Graphics
Printed in the United States of America by BookCrafters

Library of Congress Cataloging-in-Publication Data

Hegde, M. N. (Mahabalagiri, N.), 1941–
Pocketguide to treatment in speech-language pathology / M.N. Hegde.
p. cm.
Includes bibliographical references.
ISBN 1-56593-274-9
1. Speech therapy—Handbooks, manuals, etc. 2. Speech disorders—Handbooks, manuals, etc. I. Title.
[DNLM: 1. Speech-Language Pathology—handbooks. WL 39 H462p 1995]
RC423.H38288 1995
616.85'506—dc20
DNLM/DLC
for Library of Congress 95-39127
CIP

ABBREVIATED CONTENTS: ENTRIES BY DISORDERS

Preface

This PocketGuide to treatment procedures in speech-language pathology has been designed for clinical practitioners and students in communicative disorders. The PocketGuide combines the most desirable features of a specialized dictionary of terms, clinical resource book, and textbooks and manuals on treatment. It is meant to be a quick reference book like a dictionary because the entries are alphabetized; but it offers more than a dictionary because it specifies treatment procedures in a "do this" format. The PocketGuide is like a resource book in that it avoids theoretical and conceptual aspects of procedures presented; but it offers more than a resource book by clearly specifying the steps involved in treating clients. The PocketGuide is like standard textbooks that describe treatment procedures; but it organizes the information in a manner conducive to more ready use. By avoiding theoretical background and controversies, the PocketGuide gives the essence of treatment in a step-by-step form that promotes easy understanding and ready reference just before beginning treatment. The PocketGuide does not suggest that theoretical and research issues are not important in treating clients; it just assumes that the user is familiar with them.

How the PocketGuide is Organized

Each main entry is printed in bold and burgundy color. Each cross-referenced entry is underlined. Each main disorder of communication is entered in its alphabetical order. Subcategories or types of a given disorder are described under the main entry (e.g., *Broca's Aphasia* under *Aphasia*).

Specific techniques, most of them with general applicability across disorders (e.g., *Modeling, Biofeedback*, or *Turn Taking*) also are alphabetized. Such specific techniques generally are described at their main alphabetical entry (e.g., *Modeling* under M). When appropriate, the reader also is referred to the disorders for which the techniques are especially appropriate.

For most disorders, a general and composite treatment procedure is first described. For example, there is a general treatment program described for *Stuttering* or *Language Disorders in Children*. Following this description of a generic treatment procedure, specific techniques or treatment programs are described (e.g., treating auditory comprehension problems in aphasia, pragmatic problems in language disorders in children, or rate reduction in stuttering; and such treatment programs as *Helm Elicited Program for Syntax Stimulation* or the *Monterey Fluency Program*). Organization of entries varies somewhat for different disorders, but an example of a general organization used in the guide follows:

Articulation and Phonological Disorders. (Definition)
A General Articulation Treatment Procedure
Treatment of Articulation and Phonological Disorders: Specific Techniques or Programs
Behavioral Approaches
Contrast Approach
Cycles Approach
Distinctive Feature Approach
Multiple Phoneme Approach
Paired Stimuli Approach
Phonological Knowledge Approach
Phonological Process Approach
Sensory Motor Approach
Traditional Approach

Many treatment concepts and procedures are cross-referenced. All cross-referenced entries are underlined. Therefore, the reader who comes across an underlined term can look up that term in a different place or context.

How to Use This PocketGuide

There are two methods for the clinician to use this guide. In the **first method**, the clinician looks up treatment procedures by disorders in their alphabetical order; an **Abbreviated Contents: Entries by Disorders** will quickly refer the reader to specific communication disorders described in the guide. Treatment procedures of the following major disorders are described in their alphabetical order:

Aphasia
Apraxia of Speech
Articulation and Phonological Disorders
Cerebral Palsy
Cleft Palate
Cluttering
Dementias
Dysarthrias
Dysphagia
Language Disorders in Children
Laryngectomy
Right Hemisphere Syndrome
Stuttering
Traumatic Brain Injury
Voice Disorders

Under each of the main entries for major disorders, the clinician may look up subentries or specific types of disorders. For example, under **Dysarthria**, the clinician will find the following alphabetized subentries and their treatment procedures:

Ataxic Dysarthria
Flaccid Dysarthria
Hyperkinetic Dysarthria
Hypokinetic Dysarthria
Mixed Dysarthria
Spastic Dysarthria
Unilateral Upper Motor Neuron Dysarthria

In the **second method**, the clinician looks up treatment procedures by **their name**. For example the clinician can look up such specific treatment techniques as the following in their alphabetical order:

Activity-based Language Intervention
Airflow Management in Stuttering

Augmentative Communication
Behavioral Momentum
Child-Centered Approaches to Language Intervention
Collaborative Model
Conversational Repair
Delayed auditory feedback
Differential Reinforcement of Alternative Behaviors (DRA)
Environmental Language Intervention Strategy
Event Structure
Functional Equivalence Training
Joint-Action Routines
Incidental Teaching Method
Isolated Therapy Model
Mand-Model
Melodic Intonation Therapy
Narrative Skills Training
Prolonged speech
Rate Reduction in Treating Dysarthria
Whole Language Approach
and so forth

If appropriate, the reader who finds a specific treatment technique in the general alphabetized order is referred to the specific disorder for which the technique is relevant.

A Caveat

Serious attempts have been made to include most treatment techniques described in the literature. However, the author is aware that not all techniques have been included. Some have been excluded because of their transparent lack of logic, appropriateness, or even an expectation of desirable effects. A few are defined because they are popular or being advocated. However, they are not described fully because of the presence of strong negative evidence. Most importantly, in any task such as this that requires encyclopedic review of literature, omission of a procedure that deserves inclusion is an acknowledged and unintended limitation. The reader may be more often correct in assuming that a technique was omitted inadvertently than to assume that it was considered and rejected.

The author did not set for himself the impossible goal of including all treatment techniques. The practical goal was shaped more by such descriptors or qualifiers of treatment techniques as *most*, the *major*, the *generally effective*, the *most widely* practiced, and so forth. Such qualifiers necessarily involve judgment with which clinicians will disagree. If some techniques included do not meet these qualifiers, that is fine; the author would rather err in that direction. On the other hand, errors of omission are correctable through revisions. Therefore, the author is open to suggestions from clinicians and researchers.

Although most treatment techniques in communicative disorder are in need of treatment effectiveness or efficacy data, those that are especially deficient are noted in their description or definition. Those treatment techniques that have especially strong supportive evidence also are noted. In most cases, unfortunately, information on effects and efficacy is unavailable or ambiguous. This guide is not a means of evaluating treatment techniques; such evaluation is solely the responsibility of the clinician who selects treatment techniques. To help the clinician make such evaluations, procedures and experimental designs that are used in treatment efficacy research are included in this guide. Also included are suggested *Treatment Selection Criteria*.

I would like to thank Susan Atherton who has assisted me in preparing this PocketGuide. My special thanks go to Glen Tellis who has helped research the vast treatment literature. His commitment and assistance have been invaluable in completing this project.

ABA Design. A single-subject research design used to evaluate treatment effects; a target behavior is first baserated (A), taught with the procedure to be evaluated (B), and then reduced (A) by withdrawing treatment to show that the teaching was effective.

- Baserate the target behavior to be taught
- Apply the new treatment to be evaluated
- When the behavior increases, withdraw treatment
- Chart the results to show that the results for the baserate and withdrawal conditions were similar but those for the treatment condition were different.

ABAB Design. A single-subject research design used to evaluate treatment efficacy; a target behavior is first baserated (A), taught by applying the treatment program (B), reduced by withdrawing or reversing the treatment (A), and then taught again by reapplying the treatment (B) to show that the teaching was effective. The design has two versions: Reversal and Withdrawal.

- Baserate the behavior to be taught
- Apply the new treatment to be evaluated for the target behavior
- Briefly, apply treatment to another behavior or simply withdraw treatment
- Again treat the target behavior
- Chart the results to show that the two no-treatment conditions were convincingly different from the two treatment conditions.

ABAB Reversal Design. A single-subject design for evaluating treatment effects; a desirable behavior is baserated (A), taught (B), reduced by teaching its counterpart (A), and then taught again (B) to show that the teaching was effective.

- Baserate the behavior to be taught
- Apply the new treatment to be evaluated for the target behavior
- Briefly, apply treatment to an incompatible behavior
- Again treat the target behavior

- Chart the results to show that the behavior varied according to the treatment and reversal operations

ABAB Withdrawal Design. A single-subject research design for evaluating treatment effects; a desirable behavior is baserated (A), taught (B), reduced by withdrawing the treatment (A), and then taught again (B) to show that teaching was effective.

- Baserate the behavior to be taught
- Apply the new treatment to be evaluated
- When the behavior increases, withdraw treatment
- Reapply treatment
- Chart the results to show that the behavior varied according to the treatment and withdrawal operations

Hegde, M. N. (1994). *Clinical research in communicative disorders: Principles and strategies* (2nd ed.). Austin, TX: Pro-Ed.

Abduction. Separation of the vocal folds.

Adduction. Approximation of the vocal folds.

Airflow Management. A stuttering treatment target; includes inhalation of air, slight exhalation before initiating phonation, and sustained air flow throughout an utterance; for procedures see Stuttering, Treatment; Treatment of Stuttering: Specific Techniques or Programs.

Alaryngeal Speech. Speech without a biological larynx; a mode of communication for persons whose larynges have been surgically removed; may be electronically assisted, pneumatically assisted, or esophageal; for treatment procedures, see Laryngectomy.

Alerting Stimuli. Various means of drawing the client's attention to the imminent treatment stimuli; include such statements as "Get ready! Here comes the picture!" or "Look at me, I am about to show you how;" or such nonverbal cues as touching the client's hand just before presenting a stimulus.

Alphabet Board. A communication board with the alphabet printed on it; may also contain a few words and sentences; the client simultaneously speaks and points to the first letter of each spoken word printed and displayed on the board.

Alphabet Board Supplementation. A technique used in reducing the speech rate and thus improving intelligibility in clients with dysarthria; to reduce rate, the method requires clients to point to the first letter of each word on an alphabet board.

Arrange an alphabet board with large capital letters

Ask the client to point to the first letter of each word to be spoken on the board

Yorkston, K. M., Beukleman, D., & Bell, K. (1988). *Clinical management of dysarthric speakers.* San Diego, CA: College-Hill Press.

Alternative Communication. Methods of nonoral, nonvocal communication that serve as alternatives to oral speech and language; only in a few extreme cases are the methods totally alternative; most nonoral, nonvocal means of communication augment oral and vocal communication; treatment techniques described under Augmentative Communication, a term some prefer.

Alzheimer's Disease. A degenerative neurological disorder caused by Neurofibrillary Tangles, Neuritic Plaques, Granulovacuolar Degeneration, and neurochemical changes; characterized by deterioration in behavior, cognition, memory, language, communication, and personality; most common of the irreversible dementias; general management procedures described under Dementia; in addition, consider the following additional suggestions:

- Use good lighting if a visual perceptual deficit is present
- Approach the client within his or her visual field
- Teach superordinate category names (e.g., *tools* and *furniture*) instead of basic level names (e.g., *socket wrench* and

footstool) because superordinate category names appear to be relatively unaffected
- Teach compensatory strategies for lost functions
- Teach gestures as a means of communicating
- Orient the client to activities of daily living
- Use intensive auditory stimulation
- Provide new information that is an extension of the familiar
- Develop a theme for each treatment session
- Use praise that is appropriate for an adult
- Speak slowly
- Wait for a sign that the client has understood before progressing to the next topic
- Use the same spoken phrases to inform the client about routine tasks (e.g., say, "Let's go out" when it is time to go out and say "Your food is ready" when it is time to eat)

American Indian Hand Talk (AMER-IND). tem of nonverbal communication used by native Americans to communicate with members of other tribes with different languages; a manual interlanguage; the signs represent ideas and many are pictographic; gestures may be produced in series to express more complex ideas, called agglutination; many signs are one-handed; used in teaching Augmentative Communication, Gestural (Unaided).

American Sign Language (ASL or AMESLAN). A highly developed manual (gestural) language used mostly by deaf persons in the United States; a communication target for certain nonverbal or minimally verbal persons; each sign or gesture may represent a letter of the English alphabet, a word, or a phrase; signs provide phonemic, morphologic, and syntactic information; used in teaching Augmentative Communication, Gestural (Unaided).

Analogies. Logical inferences that are based on the assumption that if two things are similar in certain aspects, then they must be alike in other aspects.

Anomia. Difficulty in naming people, places, or things; a major symptom of Aphasia.

Antecedents. Events that occur before responses; stimuli or events the clinician presents in treatment. Antecedents may be:

- Objects
- Pictures
- Re-created or enacted events
- Instructions, demonstrations, modeling, prompting, manual guidance, and other special stimuli

Aphasia. A language disorder caused by brain injury in which (a) all aspects of language comprehension and production are impaired to varying degrees (a nontypological definition); (b) one or more aspects of language comprehension and language production may be affected (a typological definition).

Treatment of Aphasia, General Guidelines

- Reduce the effects of the residual deficits on the personal, emotional, social, family, and occupational aspects of the client's life
- Teach compensatory strategies
- Counsel family members to help them cope with the residual deficits
- Give a realistic prognosis that modifies the clients' and the family members' expectations
- Structure the treatment and let the client repeatedly practice the target behaviors
- Develop a variety of client-specific treatment procedures
- Exploit the client's strengths (e.g., use the stronger visual mode to supplement the weaker auditory mode)
- Judge when it is not useful or ethical to continue the treatment
- Observe the client carefully
- Conduct a detailed assessment
- Choose client-specific target behaviors that enhance functional communication
- Sequence target behaviors in treatment

- Move from simple to complex tasks
- Use extra stimulus control initially
- Use modeling, pictures, and objects
- Reduce stimulus control in small steps
- Arrange consequences that occur naturally
- Provide immediate, response-contingent feedback
- Encourage the client to self-monitor
- Train family members to evoke, prompt, reinforce, and maintain communicative behaviors

Auditory Comprehension

Factors That Promote Auditory Comprehension

- More frequently used words
- Nouns rather than verbs, adjectives, and adverbs
- Picturable verbs and other words
- Unambiguous pictures
- Shorter sentences
- Syntactically simpler sentences
- Active sentences
- Personally relevant information
- Slower speech with frequent pauses
- Slower rate with words that are stressed
- Quieter environment
- Redundant Messages
- Connected speech rather than isolated words or sentences
- Limited response choices
- Accompanied auditory stimuli with appropriate visual stimuli
- Visibility of the speaker's face
- Alerting Stimuli presented before the evoking stimulus is presented

Sequence of Auditory Comprehension Treatment

Comprehension of *Single Words*.

to:

- Body parts
- Objects
- Pictures of objects

- Clothing items
- Food items
- Action pictures

Comprehension of *Spoken Sentences*. Move from:

- Simpler sentences to more complex sentences
- More redundant to less redundant sentences
- Sentences with familiar information to those with unfamiliar information

Comprehension of *Spoken Questions*. Ask:

- Concrete yes/no questions ("Are you sitting in the wheelchair?")
- Abstract yes/no questions ("Is a plant bigger than a tree?")
- Simpler open-ended questions
- More complex open-ended questions

Comprehension of *Spoken Directions*. As the client to:

- Point to single objects or pictures (single verb)
- Point to objects in sequence ("Point to the pen and then the paper.")
- Manipulate stimuli in sequence ("Point to the pen and then lift up the paper.")
- Manipulate objects according to directions ("Put the ball in the box.")

Comprehension of *Discourse*. Target such skills as:

- Turn taking
- Topic maintenance
- Switching roles between listener and speaker (consider using the PACE program at this level)

Treatment of Aphasia: Verbal Expression

Treatment of Naming: Designing Problem-specific Strategies

Design treatment to suit the kind of anomia present:

Word production anomia: Anomia due mainly to motor problems; often does not need direct treatment; provide such simple cues as the first sound of target word.

Word selection anomia: Clients can describe, gesture, write, and draw to suggest a word they cannot say, can correctly recognize the name when given; cueing, including gestures, descriptions, and drawing is not very effective.

Semantic anomia. Patients do not recognize the words they cannot produce; train word recognition.

Limited anomia. Disconnection anomias; such category-specific problems as difficulty naming animals or vegetables; pair unimpaired skills with impaired naming.

Delayed response. Presumably due to the slow activation of the naming process; shape progressively faster reaction time.

Self-corrected errors. Prompting might be effective; reinforce self-correction.

Perseveration. Persisting errors; reduce their frequency.

Unrelated words. Irrelevant responses; reduce their frequency.

Paraphasias. Unintended word or sound substitutions; reduce their frequency by increasing the production of target words.

Treatment of Naming: General Considerations

Use stimuli that facilitate correct naming:

- High frequency words
- Names of manipulable objects
- Objects rather than pictures
- Realistic drawings rather than line or abstract drawings
- Phonemic cues
- Client-regulation of stimulus presentation
- Extra time to respond
- Longer (30 seconds or more) stimulus exposure time
- Simultaneous visual and auditory stimulus presentation

Treatment of Naming: Targets and Techniques

Confrontation Naming: Treatment Procedure:

- Place a picture or an objects in front of the client
- Ask "What is this?"
- Prompt the correct response
- Reinforce the correct response

Naming in General: Treatment Procedure:

Use cueing hierarchies (Response evoking stimuli arranged in hierarchies)

- Find a stimulus (cue) that evokes the response
- Use a stronger cue only when weaker cues do not evoke the response
- Start with a few cues and add more only when necessary
- Use different types of cues:
- Fade the cue so that natural stimuli come to evoke the response

Types of Cues

Modeling

- Ask a question ("What is this?")
- Immediately model the response ("Say, a book")
- Let the client imitate
- Reinforce the client for correct imitation

Sentence completion: Give parts of sentences as cues

Clinician (CN): "You write with a ____________?"

Client (CT): "Pen."

CN: " You write with a ball-point ____________?"

CT: "Pen."

Phonetic cues: Give initial sounds as cues

CN: "You write with a (pause); the word starts with a p_____"

CT: "Pen."

Syllabic cues: Give syllables of words as cues when the sound cue is not effective

CN: "This is a spoo___"

CT: "Spoon."

Silent phonetic cues: Give articulatory postures without vocalizations as cues

CN: "This is a ___" (silent articulatory posture for p).

CT: "Pen."

Functional descriptions as cues: Give a description of an object in terms of its use as cues

CN: "This is a round object that you roll or kick. What do you call it?"

CT: "Ball."

Description and demonstration of an action as cues: Request the target name, and describe and demonstrate an action as cues

CN: "What is this? You use this to write" (demonstrate writing).

CT: "Pen."

Client description as cues: Ask a client to first say what an object is used for and then name it

CN: "Tell me what you use this for and then tell me its name."

CT: "I use it to write. It is a pen."

Patient's demonstration of functions as cues: Ask the client to first demonstrate the function of an object and then name it

CN: "Show me how you use this and then tell me the name."

CT: Demonstrates the action of drinking and then says "cup."

Objects or pictures with their printed names as Present an object or a picture with its printed name and ask the client to name it

CN: Presents a book (or a picture of a book), the printed word book, and then asks the client, "What is this?"

CT: "Book."

Patient's oral spelling as cues: Ask the client to spell a word orally and then say the word (name).

Patient's spelling and writing as cues: Ask the client to spell a word, write it, and then say it.

Presentation of sound as a cue: Present a sound associated with an object and then ask the client to name it.

Deblocking: Direct and Indirect. Treating naming or word-finding problems in clients with aphasia by presenting a variety of stimuli to which the person can respond and then presenting the target stimulus for the client to respond to.

Direct deblocking: Presenting several unrelated words along with the target word (e.g., the clinician says several words along with "cup"; then asks the client to name the picture of a cup)

Indirect deblocking: Presenting a word typically associated with a target word and then asking the client to produce it; the clinician does not present the target word (e.g., the clinician says "woman" to evoke the word "wife").

Treatment of Functional Communication

Communication skills useful in social situations; final targets of aphasia treatment; in addition to the following generic treatment procedure, consider using one of several special programs described later in this section under Treatment of Aphasia: Specific Techniques or Programs; integrate compatible procedures.

- Target communication as opposed to linguistic accuracy as the primary target in this stage of treatment
- Select words, phrases, and sentences that are most useful:
  - for the client and his or her caregivers
  - in expressing the client's personal experiences, bodily needs, emotions, and thoughts
  - in simple, everyday social situations and conversational contexts
- Design client-specific treatment programs in which you shape progressively longer utterances
- Start with what the client can say, perhaps a few words or even syllables
- Add other syllables to create words, or words to create phrases
- Add additional words to create sentences
- Evoke a variety of sentence structures

- noun and verb combinations
- active declarative sentences
- requests, commands, demands
- wh-questions
- structures with adjectives
- structures with comparatives
- yes/no questions
- structures with prepositions, pronouns, present progressives, and so forth

- Use special stimuli that are necessary (pictures, modeling, prompting, and so forth)
- Fade the special stimuli out, and fade in the naturalistic stimuli
- Reinforce the client productions
- Move to conversational speech
  - engage the client in meaningful, functional conversation
  - ask the client to describe personal experiences, hobbies, professional experiences, family related events, favorite foods, entertainment, books read, vacations taken, and so forth
  - narrate a story and ask the client to retell it
  - role play Turn Taking
  - reinforce the client for staying on a topic; extend the duration of Topic Maintenance
- Implement a maintenance program
  - train the client to generate his or her own cues for better speech
    - teach the client to self-monitor
    - implement treatment in naturalistic settings
    - use natural response consequences
  - train health care professionals to support and socially reinforce the communicative behaviors
  - train family members to
    - evoke and reinforce speech
    - reduce demands when it is appropriate
    - pay attention to the client's strengths

- express emotional support for the client
- include the client in communicative and other social activities

Chapey, R. (1994) (Ed.). *Language intervention strategies in adult aphasia*. Baltimore, MD: Williams & Wilkins.

Davis, G. A. (1993). *A survey of adult aphasia* (2nd ed.). Englewood Cliffs, NJ: Prentice-Hall.

Hegde, M. N. (1994). *A coursebook on neurogenic language disorders*. San Diego, CA: Singular Publishing Group.

Rosenbek, J. C., LaPointe, L. L., & Wertz, R. T. (1989). *Aphasia: A clinical approach*. Austin, TX: Pro-Ed.

Treatment of Aphasia: Specific Types

Broca's Aphasia. A type of aphasia characterized by nonfluent, effortful speech with missing grammatical elements; marked difficulty in naming; slow rate of speech and limited word output; limited syntax; better auditory comprehension; may have associated dysarthria and apraxia of speech; usually associated with lesions in the third frontal convolution of the left or dominant hemisphere.

- Use procedures described under Aphasia; Treatment of Aphasia: Verbal Expression; specifically:
  - Increase length of utterances
  - Increase complexity of responses
  - Decrease grammatical errors
  - Treat naming difficulties
  - Decrease stereotypic utterances
  - Use modeling
  - Model progressively longer utterances and ask the client to imitate
  - Teach nouns and verbs on successive trials
  - Provide immediate, positive feedback
  - Ask questions to evoke responses
  - Encourage pointing, gestures, drawing, writing, and reading to improve verbal expression
  - Teach a sign language system (e.g., AMER-IND) if necessary

- Select one of the special programs described under Aphasia; Treatment of Aphasia: Special Programs (e.g., A Program of Changing Criteria, the Helm Elicited Language Program for Syntax Stimulation, or Promoting Aphasics' Communicative Effectiveness)

Global Aphasia. A type of aphasia characterized by severe deficits in comprehension and production of language; all sensory modalities may be affected; caused by widespread damage to language areas of the brain.

- Eliminate distractions
- Face the client
- Reduce your rate of speech
- Pause at syntactic junctures and between stimulus presentations
- Use appropriate stress and intonation
- Use short sentences
- Pause between sentences
- Use nonverbal cues to improve communication
- Select basic, simple, functional words and phrases for initial treatment
- Select words and phrases that express basic needs
- Accept any mode of response: verbal, gestural, or signed
- Provide both auditory and visual stimulation
- Provide multiple stimuli (modeling, pictures, written stimuli, objects, gestures)
- Begin treatment with modeling and require immediate imitation
- Ask for delayed imitation later; give the client time to respond
- Fade modeling and other additional stimuli
- Shape the response
- Provide manual guidance
- Give prompt, natural, and social reinforcement
- Teach responses to simple questions
- Teach simple requests
- Teach simple descriptions

- Move to basic conversational skills training
- Improve writing skills
- Teach gestures and consider techniques described under Augmentative Communication (including AMER-IND, Communication Boards, and Blissymbolics).
- Consider one of the special programs (Aphasia; Treatment of Aphasia: Special Programs, including Visual Action Therapy and Gestural Reorganization)
- Counsel the family about the effects of stroke, the communication problems and prospects of treatment, home strategies to enhance communication, and so forth

Collins, M. (1991). *Diagnosis and treatment of global aphasia.* San Diego: Singular Publishing Group.

Transcortical Motor Aphasia. A type of nonfluent aphasia characterized by agrammatic, paraphasic, and telegraphic speech; distinguishing feature is intact repetition; lesion is typically outside Broca's area, found often in the deep portions of the left frontal lobe or below or above Broca's area.

Use imitation and naming to improve speaking

- Select pictures as stimuli
  - ask the client to say or write nouns and verbs that the pictures suggest
  - if the client fails, point out dominant aspects of the stimulus or prompt nouns and verbs
  - obtain from the client or supply three or more words for each picture
- Ask the client to form sentences with one of the words produced or supplied
- Ask the client to expand the sentence with other words
- Reinforce all attempts in the right direction

Use relatively intact reading skills to prime or promote speaking

- Begin treatment sessions with client reading general printed materials aloud to deblock speaking

- Begin controlled conversational treatment after an extended period of reading
- Relate conversation to the reading if necessary, or unrelated if possible
- Have the client read selected utterances (prepared for the client) and then say them if general reading does not deblock speaking
- Have the client read more complex materials and answer questions about them
- Model if necessary
- Use story books with pictures, ask the client to first read the story, and then describe the pictures in the same book

Rosenbek, J. C., LaPointe, L. L., & Wertz, R. T. (1989). *Aphasia: A clinical approach*. Austin, TX: Pro-Ed.

Wernicke's Aphasia. A type of fluent aphasia characterized by good or even excessive fluency of speech, rapid rate, normal articulation and prosody, good grammatical structures, paraphasia, neologism, jargon, and generally meaningless speech; poor auditory comprehension is a major distinguishing feature; the lesion is in Wernicke's area.

- Reduce the impulsive and incessant talking:
  - structure the treatment sessions and reduce distracting stimuli
  - ask the client to listen
  - use gestures and manual guidance to stop the client from talking (touch your lips with your index finger to suggest "be quiet," touch the client's hand to make him or her to stop talking)
  - ask yes/no questions and accept only such answers, not elaborate utterances
- Expand utterances in a controlled manner
- Treat auditory comprehension deficits; use relevant procedures described under Aphasia; Treatment of Aphasia (especially the guidelines and procedures described under Auditory Comprehension)

- Use one of the special programs described under Aphasia; Treatment of Aphasia: Special Techniques or Programs, including Treatment for Wernicke's Aphasia (TWA)

Treatment of Aphasia: Specific Techniques or Programs

Gestural Reorganization. A method of teaching verbal expression by first pairing them with gestures and then fading the gestures; described by J. Rosenbek, L. LaPointe, and R. Wertz.

- Select phrases or sentences for training
- Select gestures that mean the same as those target expressions
  - use gestures from American Indian Hand Talk (AMER-IND) or other systems
  - invent gestures that are appropriate for the expressions
  - explain the gestures and the treatment approach to the client
- Teach the gestures to the client
  - ask the client to match your gesture
  - ask the client to match pictures of gestures
  - teach functional and spontaneous use of gestures
- Combine the learned gestures with speaking (verbal expression)
  - model the gesture and the verbal expression
  - model only one of them
  - use Manual Guidance if necessary (manually help form the gesture)
  - have the client practice the two separately, only if necessary; combine them
- Fade the gestures and continue to evoke and reinforce the verbal expressions

Rosenbek, J. C., LaPointe, L. L., & Wertz, R. T. (1989). *Aphasia: A clinical approach*. Austin, TX: Pro-Ed.

Helm Elicited Program for Syntax Stimulation. An aphasia treatment program designed to increase the production of syntactically correct utterances in agrammatic clients with moderate to well-preserved auditory comprehension and some speech production; developed by N. Helm-Estabrooks; uses pictures and a story completion method to evoke the following 11 sentence types at two levels (Level A and Level B):

1. Imperative Intransitive ("Lie down")
2. Imperative Transitive ("Wash the dishes")
3. Wh-interrogative ("What are you doing?")
4. Declarative Transitive ("She cleans teeth")
5. Declarative Intransitive ("She skates")
6. Comparative ("They're funnier")
7. Passive ("The suitcases were lost")
8. Yes/No Questions ("Did you buy the paper?")
9. Direct and Indirect Object ("They give Pat a cake")
10. Embedded Sentences ("She wanted him to be healthy")
11. Future ("He will hike")

Background and Preparation

- Obtain the entire treatment program or prepare your own questions, stories, and pictures
- Baserate the responses

Level A

- Select sentence type 1.
- Read a story containing a target sentence; ask the client to produce the target sentence:

  Clinician (CN): "My friend feels dizzy, so I tell him, 'lie down.' What do I tell him?"

  Client (CT): "Lie down."

- Upon reaching a 90% accuracy criterion, move to Level B.

Level B

- Read a short story again, but without the target sentence; ask the client to produce the target sentence:

  CN: "My friend feels dizzy, so I tell him what?"

  CT: "Lie down."

- Upon reaching 90% accuracy criterion for sentence type I at Level B, select sentence type 2 for training;

use the same procedure as for sentence type 1.

- Complete training on all 11 sentence types

Helm-Estabrooks, N. (1981. *Helm elicited program for syntax stimulation*. Austin, TX: PRO-ED.

Helm-Estabrooks, N., & Albert, M. L. (1991). *Manual of aphasia therapy*. Austin, TX: PRO-ED.

Melodic Intonation Therapy (MIT). An aphasia treatment program for clients with severe nonfluent aphasia with good auditory comprehension; developed by M. Albert, R. Sparks, and N. Helm; uses musical intonation, continuous voicing, and rhythmic tapping to teach verbal expression; hierarchically structured; contraindicated for clients with Wernicke's, transcortical motor or sensory, and global aphasia; has three levels.

General Procedures

- Select high probability words, phrases, and sentences
- Use pictures or environmental cues for each target utterance
- Intone each word, phrase, or sentence slowly and with constant voicing
- Maintain pitch and stress variations of normal speech
- Tap the client's left hand once for each intoned syllable
- Signal with your left hand when to listen and when to intone
- Generally, move to the earlier step when the client fails at a step

Level I

- Humming: Show a picture, hum the target item, and tap; no response required
- Unison singing: Intone in unison with the client and tap
- Unison with fading: Intone, tap, and fade halfway through the phrase
- Immediate repetition: Ask the client to listen to you as you intone the phrase and tap; let the client imitate
- Response to a probe question: Following a correct imitation, intone a probe question (e.g., "What did you say?")

Level II

- Introduction of item: Intone the phrase twice and tap; no response required
- Unison with fading: Intone, tap, and fade halfway through the phrase
- Delayed repetition: Intone and tap, and after 6 seconds of delay, let the client tap with assistance; ask the client to intone without help
- Response to a probe question: Six seconds following the client's response, intone the probe question; do not hand tap; let the client intone the phrase

Level III

- Delayed repetition: Tap and intone and let the client intone the phrase after 6 seconds and give tapping assistance
- Introducing *sprechgesang* (speech song). Present the target phrase twice slowly, without singing, but with exaggerated rhythm and stress; no tapping and no response required
- Delayed spoken repetition. Present the phrase in normal prosody, without hand tapping and let the client imitate after 6 seconds in normal prosody
- Response to a probe question. Ask a probe question with normal prosody after a 6-second delay; let the client respond with normal prosody

Albert, M., Sparks, R., & Helm, N. (1973). Melodic intonation therapy for aphasia. *Archives of Neurology, 29*, 130–131.

Helm-Estabrooks, N., Nicholas, M., & Morgan, A. (1989). *Melodic intonation therapy program.* San Antonio, TX: Special Press. *See this source for a complete description of steps, scoring procedure, and stimulus materials.*

Program of Changing Criteria. An aphasia treatment program described by J. Rosenbek, L. LaPointe, and R. Wertz to increase the length and quality of language; uses systematic shaping and progressively higher response criteria requiring longer utterances; uses differential reinforcement and extensive practice.

- Select realistic human action pictures to evoke responses
- Write about 10 questions some of which you will use with each picture (e.g., "How many people do you see?"; "What are they doing?"; "What is the person wearing"?)
- Begin at Criterion I. Require a one- or two-word response
  - give directions, present a picture, and ask a question
  - if no or incorrect response, use the Cloze Procedure
  - if the client fails, model the response
  - if the client fails, use any other procedure to evoke the response
  - if the client fails, use another program
  - reinforce and give repeated practice on correct responses
- Move to Criterion II. Require a three- to five-word response
  - give cloze-like cues when the response is incorrect
  - if the client fails, model the correct response
  - if no imitation, use any other method to evoke the response
  - if still no success, return to Criterion I or shift to another program
  - reinforce and give repeated practice on correct responses
- Move to Criterion III. Require six- to eight-word responses; use the same procedures as under Criterion II.
- Move to Criterion IV. Require spontaneous description of pictures with sentences containing nine or more words; but be flexible about this to promote natural productions.

Rosenbek, J. C., LaPointe, L. L., & Wertz, R. T. (1989). *Aphasia: A clinical approach*. Austin, TX: Pro-Ed.

Promoting Aphasics' Communicative Effectiveness An aphasia treatment program designed to promote face-to-face conversation; developed by G. A. Davis and J. Wilcox; emphasis on exchange of new information, functional communication (as against linguistic precision) with turn taking, free choice for the client to communicate in any modality; and natural feedback.

- Use a large number of stimulus cards that contain pictured objects, actions, and stories; stack the cards face down on the table
- Take turns drawing cards from the stack; communicate information about the stimulus
- Encourage any mode of expression (words, gestures, drawings, writing, pointing, or a combination of these)
- Add new stimulus cards to promote the exchange of new information
- Provide natural consequences (e.g., What did you say? Do you mean________? I am not sure . . .)
- Acknowledge the client's message while suggesting the correct word or words (e.g., "I understand. You mean *book*, right?")
- Make variations and adaptations
- Exchange the roles of speaker and listener with the client

Davis, G. A. (1993). *A survey of adult aphasia* (2nd ed.). Englewood Cliffs, NJ: Prentice-Hall.

Response Elaboration Training. A treatment approach that uses a loose training format; designed to expand utterances of aphasic clients; emphasis is on shaping and chaining client- rather than clinician-initiated utterances; allows a wide variety of responses as against a predetermined correct response; developed and researched by K. Kearns and his associates.

- Select line drawings to stimulate speech
- Show a stimulus card and evoke an initial response, any response (e.g., the client may say "Man . . . sweeping" to a line drawing of a person with a broom)
- Reinforce the client; also, shape and model the client's response (e.g., say, "Great. The man is sweeping")
- Ask a *Wh*-question to evoke an elaboration of the initial utterance (e.g., ask "Why is he sweeping?")
- Reinforce the client's elaboration and shape and model the initial response combined with the subsequent elaboration (e.g., the client may answer by saying "wife . . .

mad" and you say, "Way to go! The man is sweeping the floor because his wife is mad")

- Model the longer response a second time and ask the client to "Try and say the whole thing after me. Say . . .")
- Ask the client to imitate after a delay if the client is successful at the previous step
- Continue until the client fails to elaborate any more
- Introduce another picture for a similar sequence or initiate a different initial response for the same picture

Kearns, K. P., & Scher, G. P. (1989). The generalization of response elaboration training effects. In T. E. Prescott (Ed.), *Clinical Aphasiology* (Vol. 18, pp. 223–245). Austin, TX: Pro-Ed.

Schuell's Auditory Stimulation Approach for Aphasia. The method concentrates on intensive auditory stimulation or auditory bombardment; developed by H. Schuell; the method needs more clinical efficacy data.

- Find varied and abundant stimulus materials
- Design a sequence of auditory stimulation
- Work systematically and intensively
- Begin with easy and familiar tasks and increase their complexity; ask the client to:
  - point to objects named, described, spelled, and so forth
  - follow directions (simpler to more complex)
  - answer yes/no questions
  - respond to alternate items (switch responses) (e.g., "Show me the horse/Tell me your name.")
  - repeat words, phrases, and sentences
  - complete your sentences
  - answer different kinds of questions
  - form simple sentences
  - retell stories
  - describe pictures and events
  - engage in conversation
  - copy and write words
- Provide intensive auditory stimulation
- Combine auditory stimulation with visual stimulation

- Elicit responses to each stimulation, but do not force them
- Elicit many and varied responses
- Do not correct responses; instead repeat stimulation
- Give such feedback as visual charting of progress made in treatment sessions
- Introduce new materials that contain or extend old materials

Duffy, J. R. (1994). Schuell's stimulation approach to rehabilitation. In R. Chapey (Ed.), *Language intervention strategies in adult aphasia* (3rd ed., pp. 146–174). Baltimore, MD: Williams & Wilkins.

Treatment for Wernicke's Aphasia (TWA). A method of aphasia treatment developed by N. Helm-Estabrooks and P. Fitzpatrick to treat auditory comprehension problems; appropriate for clients with severe Wernicke's aphasia who can read and understand single picturable words:

- Select a corpus of words printed in lower case that the client can read aloud and point to pictured stimuli
- Provide a printed word that the client can read, but cannot point to when named
- Ask the client to match the printed word to the picture depicting the word
- Ask the client to read the word aloud
- Ask the client to repeat the word "chair" as you say it without showing the picture
- Ask the client to point to the picture of a chair placed among other pictures
- Introduce new words as the client shows progress
- If new words cannot be introduced by about the fifth session, reevaluate the procedure; select another procedure
- Chart correct and incorrect responses on a recording sheet

Helm-Estabrooks, N., & Albert, M. L. (1991). *A manual of aphasia therapy*. Austin, TX: Pro-Ed.

Visual Action Therapy (VAT). A nonvocal, visual/gestural communication approach to the rehabilitation of globally aphasic clients; developed by N. Helm-Estabrooks and her associates; neither the clinician nor the client talk during treatment; a client who cannot match an object with the tracing of that object is not a good candidate for VAT; more treatment efficacy data are needed.

- Select 7 real objects, shaded line drawings of the objects, and seven action pictures involving the objects
- Select some contextual props (e.g., a screw in a block of wood to use a screw driver)

Level I

1. Matching pictures and objects
   - Placing objects on pictures. Place all 7 line drawings of the objects on the table; give each object to the client and gesture to place it on the correct drawing
   - Placing pictures on objects. Arrange objects on table, and ask the client to place the picture on the object
   - Pointing to objects. Rearrange objects on table, show a picture one at a time, and gesture the client to point to the object the picture represents
   - Pointing to the pictures. Rearrange pictures, show one object at a time, and gesture the client to point to the correct picture
2. Object use training
   - Pick up each object separately
   - Use props; demonstrate its use
   - Place it back on the table
   - Ask the client to pick it up and demonstrate its use
3. Action picture demonstration
   - Place an object and its corresponding action picture in front of the client
   - Point to the picture
   - Pick up the object and demonstrate its use
4. Following action picture commands
   - Place all objects and props on the table
   - Hold up an action picture
   - Gesture the client to manipulate the corresponding object

5. Pantomimed gesture demonstration
   - Place each object on the table
   - Demonstrate a gesture that represents the object; do not use props from this step on
6. Pantomimed gesture recognition
   - Produce a pantomimed gesture to represent one of the objects on the table
   - Gesture the client to point to the corresponding object
7. Pantomimed gesture production
   - Show one object at a time
   - Gesture the client to produce a gesture that suggests the object
8. Representation of hidden objects demonstration
   - Demonstrate a gesture each for two objects
   - Hide the objects in a box
   - Take one object out and gesture the hidden object.
9. Production of gestures for hidden objects
   - Have the client gesture for two objects
   - Hide them
   - Take one object out and suggest that the client gesture for the hidden object.

Level II

- Do not use objects; replace objects with action pictures beginning with Step 5 of level I

Level III

- Use only the drawings; begin with Step 5.

Helm-Estabrooks, N., & Albert, M. L. (1991). *A manual of aphasia therapy*. Austin, TX: Pro-Ed.

Aphonia. Loss of voice; a voice disorder.

Apraxia. Disordered volitional movement in the absence of muscle weakness, paralysis, or fatigue.

Apraxia of Speech (AOS) in Adults. A neurogenic speech disorder with documented neuropathology in the left cerebral hemisphere including such areas as Broca's and supplementary motor; primarily an articulatory (phonologic) disorder characterized by sensorimotor problems in positioning and sequentially moving muscles for the volitional production of speech; associated with prosodic problems; not caused by muscle weakness or neuromuscular slowness; presumed to be a disorder of motor programming for speech.

Treatment of Apraxia: General Considerations

- Start management early
- Hold frequent treatment sessions
- Consider associated problems: aphasia, dysarthria, or both
- Defer treatment for AOS until treatment for a severe aphasia produces some language production
- Organize sessions to move from easy to difficult task
- End sessions with success
- Be aware that treatment of AOS is essentially behavioral
- Be aware that prosthetic and medical management of AOS is limited and effects may be indirect and temporary
- Be aware that available data do not support the use of delayed auditory feedback in treating AOS
- Emphasize communicative efficiency and naturalness as you would with most clients in communicative disorders
- Emphasize articulatory accuracy
- Carefully sequence the speech tasks; train:
  - automatic speech before spontaneous speech
  - frequently occurring sounds before less frequently occurring sounds
  - stimulable sounds before nonstimulable sounds
  - sounds in word-initial positions before those in other positions
  - visible before nonvisible sounds
  - oral-nasal distinctions before voicing distinctions
  - voicing distinctions before manner distinctions
  - manner distinctions before place distinctions
  - bilabial and lingua-alveolar sounds before others
  - singletons before clusters
  - high-frequency words before low-frequency words

- meaningful words
- single-syllable words before multisyllable words
- single words before phrases or sentences

Treatment: General Procedures

- Provide counseling and support for the client and family
- Use consistent and variable practice
- Model sound productions frequently for the patient to imitate
- Provide systematic practice in producing the target speech sounds (drill)
- Reduce speech rate initially
- Increase speech rate as articulatory accuracy improves and stabilizes
- Use shaping to promote natural prosody
- Use phonetic placement and Phonetic Derivation
- Use a variety of sounds and sound combinations
- Practice sound productions with meaningful material
- Provide instruction on and demonstration of speech production
- Provide immediate, specific feedback
- Use instrumental feedback or biofeedback, when appropriate
- Focus treatment activities on speech tasks
- Use contrastive stress tasks
- Use the Key Word technique
- Use cueing techniques
- Use phonetic contrasts
- Use automatic speech tasks initially to evoke speech
- Use carrier phrases
- Use singing
- Push on abdomen to achieve vocal fold closure and phonation for the speechless client
- Employ an artificial larynx for the speechless patient
- Emphasize total communication (combined use of verbal expressions, gestures, writing, augmentative devices)
- Teach Self-Control (Self-Monitoring) skills:
- Use techniques of treating Articulation and Phonological Disorders

Brookshire, R. H. (1992). *An introduction to neurogenic communication disorders* (4th ed.). St. Louis, MO: Mosby Year Book.

Duffy, J. R. (1995). *Motor speech disorders: Substrates, differential diagnosis, and management*. St. Louis, MO: C. V. Mosby.

Johns, D. F. (Ed.), *Clinical management of neurogenic communicative disorders* (2nd ed.). Boston: Little, Brown

Wertz, R. T., LaPointe, L. L., & Rosenbek, J. C. (1991). *Apraxia of speech*. San Diego: Singular Publishing Group.

Treatment of Mild Apraxia

- Counsel the patient and the family; tell them about the good prospects of recovered or vastly improved communication
- Keep the focus on articulatory accuracy
- Model sound productions in words, phrases, and sentences for the client to imitate
- Require immediate imitation because it is easier than delayed imitation
- Reduce the client's rate of speech
- Use visible and simple utterances in the beginning
- Extend treatment to utterances that are more complex and sound productions that are less visible in carefully graded steps
- Use the Phonetic Placement Method
- Use Contrastive Stress Drills to promote articulatory proficiency and prosodic features of speech; in constructing contrastive drill materials:
    - use a single sound target initially in any phrase or sentence
    - use simpler and more familiar sounds initially
    - use shorter phrases or sentences initially
    - use longer words and sentences subsequently
    - add more sound targets to each utterance
    - use infrequently occurring words later
    - increase rate of speech
- Encourage the patient to create original sentences
- Ask open-ended questions
- Encourage the patient to ask questions to practice normal rhythm
- Encourage the patient to read aloud and self-correct mistakes
- Improve ability to talk under stress or interference

- Encourage self-correction
- Increase speed of response

Wertz, R. T., LaPointe, L. L., & Rosenbek, J. C. (1991). *Apraxia of speech in adults: The disorder and its management.* San Diego, CA: Singular Publishing Group.

Treatment of Moderate Apraxia

- Counsel the patient and the family about:
  - variability in symptoms
  - faster recovery of speech during the earlier weeks and slower recovery later
  - prospects for improved communication
  - potential need for long-term speech treatment
  - need to work hard in treatment
  - coping strategies
- Encourage the patient to make decisions about the future (returning to work, changing assignments at work, driving, and so forth)
- Use modeling to promote imitation of carefully selected speech sound contrasts
  - provide patients with auditory and visual cues
  - ask the patient to imitate a model
  - place a single target in varied linguistic contexts (e.g., for the target /t/, a typical list of stimuli might be *"tea, tie, toe,"* and *"two"*)
  - ask the patient to contrast the target with other sounds
  - replace single-syllable words with polysyllabic ones
  - construct phrases and sentences out of practiced words for more practice
  - make contrasts harder
  - use slow rate initially with difficult targets
  - use varying rhythm and stress (e.g., begin with equal and even stress and progress toward normal)
  - use multiple contrasts
  - encourage greater independence
  - use contrastive stress drills

- Use imitation initially
- Use a question-and-answer dialogue

Use reading in treatment

- Ask the client to read aloud
- Fade the printed stimuli by having the client:
    - look at the text and talk about it
    - look at the text and waiting before talking about it
- Teach the client to self-monitor rate, rhythm, stress, and errors

Use gestural reorganization to improve communication

- Explain the need and usefulness of Gestural Reorganization (described under Aphasia; Treatment of Aphasia: Special Techniques or Programs) to the client
- Begin with frequently used and simpler gestures (tapping with a finger, drumming with one or more fingers, squeezing the thumb and the index finger, tapping with the foot)
- Model the gesture that works for the client and ask the client to imitate
- Give Manual Guidance (e.g., physical assistance in tapping) if the client needs it
- Tap on the client's hand if this helps
- Give verbal modeling and other cues as well
- Stabilize the gesture
- Model gestures with speech and ask the patient to imitate both
- Pair gestures with words or phrases initially and pair longer utterances subsequently
- Fade your tapping first
- Fade your verbal modeling
- Use gestures with Contrastive Stress Drills
- Move on to more spontaneous conversational speech
- Fade the client's gestures if they persist as the client becomes verbally more proficient
- Use a pacing board

Wertz, R. T., LaPointe, L. L., & Rosenbek, J. C. (1991). *Apraxia of speech in adults: The disorder and its management.* San Diego, CA: Singular Publishing Group.

Treatment of Severe Apraxia

- Counsel the family members and the patient
  - give the family a reasonable statement of prognosis
  - discuss the severity of accompanying aphasia and how it might complicate apraxia treatment
  - ask the family members and health care workers to speak slowly, use shorter sentences, reduce background noise, talk only when the client is focused, and use Total Communication
  - teach family members and health care staff to use various prompts (cues) including the use of the Cloze Procedure, suggesting the first letter of the word, the first syllable of a word, paraphrasing what the client may have said for the client to indicate yes or no, and so forth.
  - ask the family and the patient to allow for some failures
  - ask the family to observe treatment and learn from it
  - tell the client what the family members are asked to do and what he or she can expect from treatment and with what efforts
- Educate the other members of the team about the client's communication problems, strengths, and the treatment program
- Begin direct treatment with modeling and ask the client to imitate; be aware that it may not work very well with severely apraxic clients who tend to perseverate
- Use the Phonetic Placement Method to help improve articulatory accuracy; encourage the client to
  - use manner distinctions (especially plosive and fricative)
  - use simultaneous manner and place distinctions
  - make voicing distinctions (evoke any kind of sound including humming or grunting and then shape it)
  - make oral-nasal distinctions
- Use Phonetic Derivation (shaping or progressive approximation) if other techniques fail

- Combine modeling, phonetic placement, and shaping (phonetic derivation) techniques
- Use rhythm to evoke speech sounds, syllables, and words; use aspects of Melodic Intonation Therapy described under Aphasia; Treatment of Aphasia: Specific Techniques or Programs
- Use the Key Word technique to have the client practice correct articulation
- For the most severely apraxic, consider using Augmentative Communication techniques

Wertz, R. T., LaPointe, L. L., & Rosenbek, J. C. (1991). *Apraxia of speech in adults: The disorder and its management.* San Diego, CA: Singular Publishing Group.

Articulation and Phonological Disorders. Disorders of speech characterized by difficulty in producing speech sounds correctly; sounds may be omitted, distorted, or substituted; difficulty in producing a few sounds with no pattern or derivable rule is often described as an articulation disorder; multiple errors that can be grouped on some principle or characteristics and thus form patterns are typically described as Phonological Disorders.

A General Articulation Treatment Procedure

- Assess the client's articulation and phonological skills; determine any patterns that may exist (based on distinctive features or phonological processes)
- Select the target speech sounds for modification; group them according to distinctive features or phonological processes, if appropriate
- Prepare stimulus materials (pictures, drawings, objects, words, phrases, and sentences)
- Establish Baselines of target sounds in words, phrases, and sentences
- Write training and probe criteria such as the following:
  - *Training Criterion*: Ninety percent (90%) accuracy in the production of sounds under training at the word level on three consecutive trials or on a set of 10 words

- *Probe Criterion*: Ninety percent (90%) accuracy in the production of sounds in untrained words presented on a series of Probe trials with at least 10 untrained words
- Train sounds at the word (or syllable) level
  - use Instructions, Demonstrations, Modeling, Shaping, and Phonetic Placement or Manual Guidance
  - organize training stimuli and their presentations, if appropriate, according to the Contrast Approach or Paired-Stimuli Approach (described later under Treatment of Articulation and Phonological Disorders: Specific Techniques or Programs)
- Use the Multiple Phoneme Approach (described later under Treatment of Articulation and Phonological Disorders: Specific Techniques or Programs) if the client can be efficiently trained with several phonemes at the same time
- Reinforcer the correct responses
- Use Corrective Feedback for incorrect responses; use verbal "No," Time-Out, or Response Cost.
- When the client meets the training criterion for a few words (4 to 6), probe for Generalized Production
  - use the Intermixed Probes procedure; alternate trained and untrained words during the probe
  - evaluate if the sounds within the pattern have changed if a pattern analysis was used (based on distinctive features or phonological processes)
- If the client meets the probe criterion, shift training to the next level of Response Complexity (from syllables to words, words to phrases, phrases to sentences)
- Select other individual sounds, distinctive features, or phonological processes for training; follow the same sequence of training and probing
- Always train the correct production of sounds in sentences and in naturalistic conversational speech
- Conduct informal training sessions in Extraclinical Settings
- Train family members, teachers, and peers in reinforcing the correct production of sounds in Natural Settings

- Teach the client Self-Control (Self-Monitoring) techniques to self-manage correct and incorrect productions
- Follow-up and provide booster treatment when the correct production in conversational speech falls below 90% accuracy

Treatment of Articulation and Phonological Disorders: Specific Techniques or Programs

Behavioral Approaches. Articulation treatment techniques based on the use of Behavioral Contingencies of stimulus-response-consequence in shaping or teaching sound production in words, sentences, and conversational speech; also may use a programmed learning approach; elements of behavioral approaches are found in almost all programs of articulation and phonological treatment including those that that are not typically described as behavioral.

Programmed Conditioning for Articulation. A behavioral treatment method that uses behavioral principles and programmed learning concepts; developed by R. Baker and B. Ryan.

- Criterion of Performance: Ten correct responses in a row.

Establishment Phase: Training Sequence:

Sound in isolation

- Sound in isolation with Continuous Reinforcement (crf)

Nonsense syllable Level

- Sound in initial position of nonsense syllables (crf)
- Sound in final position of nonsense syllables (crf)
- Sound in medial position of nonsense syllables (crf)

Word Level

- Sound in word-initial position (50% rf)
- Sound in word-final position (50% rf)
- Sound in word-medial position (50% rf)

Phrase Level

- Sound in word-initial position produced in two- or three-word phrases (50% rf)
- Sound in word-final position produced in two- or three-word phrases (50% rf)
- Sound in word-medial position produced in two- or three-word phrases (50% rf)

Sentence Level

- Sound in word-initial position produced in four- to six-word sentences (50% rf)
- Sound in word-final position produced in four- or six-word sentences (50% rf)
- Sound in word-medial position produced in four- to six-word sentences (50% rf)

Contextual Reading Level

(Go to the next level if the client is a nonreader)

- Sound in orally read sentences (crf)

Story Narration Level

- Sound in story retelling (after silently reading a story) (crf)

Picture Description Level

- Sound in sentences and phrases produced to describe a story (crf)

Conversational Speech Level

- Sound in conversational speech (crf)
- Sound in conversational speech (10% rf)

Administer the criterion test

Move to the Transfer Phase and begin training on new sounds

Transfer Phase: Training Sequence:

Home Training

Sound in words, repeats the words (crf)

- Sound in phrases, repeats the phrases (crf)
- Sound in sentences, repeats the sentences (crf)
- Sound in oral reading or picture description (crf)
- Sound in conversation (crf)

Clinician Training in Different Settings

- Conversation outside the clinic room door (crf)
- Conversation down the hall (crf)
- Conversation outside the clinic building or in another room (crf)
- Conversation in playground, cafeteria, or away from school or clinic (crf)
- Conversation outside classroom (crf)

Training in Classroom

- Conversation with clinician in classroom (crf)
- Conversation with clinician and teacher in classroom (crf)
- Conversation in small-group activity (crf)
- Conversation in large-group activity (crf)
- Speech or "show and tell" in front of the class (crf)

Administer the transfer criterion test

Maintenance Phase: Training Sequence

- Conversation during weekly meetings for the first four weeks (crf)
- Conversation during one monthly meeting (crf)
- Dismiss the client

Baker, R. D., & Ryan, B. P. (1971). *Programmed conditioning for articulation.* Monterey, CA: Monterey Learning Systems.

Contrast Approach. A cognitive-linguistic approach to treatment of articulation disorders; often used in remediating phonological processes; uses contrasting pairs of words that contain **minimal** or **maximal** differences between the target sounds and those contrasted; the actual training of sounds may involve behavioral contingencies; researched by multiple investigators.

Minimal Pair Contrast Method: Uses word pairs that have minimal phonemic contrast (e.g., *b*at-*p*at).

- Analyze the client's misarticulations
- Write minimal contrast word pairs:
- For instance, to remediate deletion of final consonants, write such pairs as *boat-bow*, *bee-bead*, and *tee-teeth*; to remediate fronting, write such pairs as *can-tan*, *key-tea*, and *gate-date*.
- Obtain pictures for words in selected pairs
- Begin treatment by modeling both the target and the contrast words; ask the child to imitate both
- Provide extensive trials on imitative production of the target and contrast words

- Ask the client to spontaneously name the picture pairs
- Ask the client to name the pictures and then sort them into separate piles
- Alternatively, ask the client to say the target word as you pick the correct picture (the client says *boat* and you pick up the picture of *boat*; if the client says *bow*, you pick-up the picture of *bow* and then correct the client)
- Ask the client to match two pictures by first picking a picture from several displayed and then selecting its minimal pair match

Maximal Pair Contrast Method. Uses word pairs that have multiple (maximal) phonemic contrasts or maximal opposition.

- Select word pairs that contrast maximally
  For instance, select such word pairs as *ch*ain-*m*ain; *c*an-*m*an; *g*ear-*f*ear (the initial phoneme in the first word of each pair is the target of treatment; the initial phoneme in the second word in each pair is the phoneme with maximal opposition)
- Use the general procedure outlined for Minimal Pair Contrast Method

Cycles Approach

A phonological pattern approach designed to treat children with multiple misarticulations and highly unintelligible speech; approach consists of treatment cycles which vary between 5 weeks and 16 weeks; includes auditory stimulation and production practices; developed by B. Hodson and E. Paden.

- Assess the client's phonological performance with 50 spontaneous naming responses and continuous speech samples; may use Hodson's *Assessment of Phonological Processes—Revised*
- Arrange a hierarchy of stimulable phonological patterns that occur in at least 40% of the relevant contexts
- Treat the most stimulable pattern first, then the next most stimulable pattern, and so on

- Target only one phonological pattern in any single session
- Treat each phoneme within a target pattern for about 60 minutes per cycle (one 60-minute, two 30-minute, or three 20-minute sessions) before moving to other phonemes within the pattern or to other patterns
- Review the prior week's production practice word cards *(see below)*; skip this step if introducing a new pattern for treatment
- Begin treatment with auditory bombardment:
  - ask the client to listen attentively for about 2 minutes as you produce 12 words with the target sound and sentences containing those words
  - slightly amplify your presentation with an auditory trainer
  - do not ask the client to produce the sounds
  - periodically contrast the correct and the incorrect production of the target sound
- Use 5 production-practice word cards: Ask the client to first say a target word and then draw, color, or paste the picture of the word on 5 × 8 index cards; write the word on the card
- Begin production practice:
  - ask the client to name about 5 target pictures (5 words per sound)
  - model the target word; use auditory, tactual, and visual cues
  - engage the client in conversation
  - use a game format
- Probe for stimulability of next session's target sounds
- Repeat the amplified auditory bombardment; present the same 12 words as before
- Ask the family members or teachers to read the same 12-word list to the client; ask the client to name the 5 picture cards used in production practice during the week
- Recycle a pattern that persists in conversational speech

Hodson, B., & Paden, E. (1983). *Targeting intelligible speech: A phonological approach to remediation.* San Diego, CA: College-Hill Press.

Distinctive Feature Approach. Articulation treatment approach based on a distinctive feature analysis; the goal is to establish missing Distinctive Features or feature contrasts by teaching relevant sounds; technically, not a treatment procedure; approach assumes that teaching a feature in the context of a few sounds will result in generalized production of other sounds with the same feature or features; more research is needed to fully support this assumption; approach is most useful with children who have multiple misarticulations that can be grouped on the basis of distinctive features; not useful for (a) treating distorted sounds as the analysis is not relevant to such errors; (b) treating a client with only a few errors that do not form patterns based on distinctive features; developed and researched by multiple investigators.

- Obtain an extended conversational speech sample
- Determine omitted and substituted sounds (phonemes in error)
- Score the distinctive features for all phonemes by assigning plus and minus values
- Select target features for treatment: select the features that are not produced at all (100% error rate) or those that have high error rate
- Select the phonemes that represent those features for teaching
- Use the programmed approach of teaching the selected sounds at the level of isolated production and production of sounds in syllables, words, phrases, and sentences
- At all levels, except for the sentence level, model the correct production for the child to imitate
- Fade modeling when the client's imitative responses are consistent
- Probe untreated sounds that share the same features as the target sounds to see if generalized productions occur
- Select additional sounds for training when there is no generalized production

- Select new sounds that contain other target features for training when there is generalized production
- Shift treatment to conversational speech inside and outside the clinic and to speech produced in home, school, and other nonclinical settings
- Teach self-monitoring
- Teach family members to praise the client for correct productions

Costello, J. M., & Onstein, J. (1976). The modification of multiple articulation errors based on distinctive feature theory. *Journal of Speech and Hearing Disorders, 41*, 199–215.

McReynolds, L. V., & Bennet, S. (1972). Distinctive feature generalization in articulation training. *Journal of Speech and Hearing Disorders, 37*, 462–470.

Multiple Phoneme Approach A method of articulation remediation in which all errors are treated in all sessions; appropriate for children with 6 or more errors; based on behavioral principles; focuses on sound production in conversational speech; does not emphasize auditory discrimination training; consists of establishment, transfer, and maintenance phases; each phase has several steps; highly structured and carefully sequenced; developed and researched by R. McCabe and D. Bradley.

- Obtain conversational speech sample of about 150 words
- Mark each word that contains at least one error
- Calculate percentage of words spoken correctly (Whole Word Accuracy: WWA)
- Use WWA measure to supplement single-word articulation tests

Phase I, Step 1. Establishment. Goal: Production of consonants in response to a printed letter or phonetic symbol representing it.

- Show an upper or lower case letter and ask "Do you know what sound this letter makes?" (visual cue only)
  - Ask the client to produce the sound in isolation on five successive trials (record the correct responses)

- If the client cannot do this, record the error and move to the next step
- Give verbal instructions along with auditory and tactile stimuli; use any other effective procedure (auditory, visual, and phonetic-placement); continue until 4 out of 5 attempts are correct; move to the next step
- Show the letter and model the sound for the child to imitate (auditory and visual stimuli only); seek 5 consecutively correct responses; then, move to the next step
- Present only the letter (visual stimulus only); ask the client to make the sound; seek 5 consecutively correct responses
  (Skip *visual only step* for children under age 5)
- In the first session or two, include sounds produced correctly to give experience of success; omit these sounds in subsequent sessions
- Reinforce correct responses (verbal praise, tokens)

Phase 1, Step 2. Holding Procedure

Designed to maintain the correct production of sounds produced in isolation when they are not yet advanced to syllable or word levels; other sounds are moved to these higher levels.

- Evoke one correct response by showing the letter once and asking the client to produce the sound (visual stimulus only)

Phase II. Transfer: Goal: Production of all target sounds in conversational speech; simultaneous training of five or more sounds; sounds may be at different levels.

Phase II, Step 1: Syllable. Used only when the client fails to produce the sound correctly in 6 out of 10 probe words (5 words with the sound in the initial position and 5 words with the sound in the final position)

- Provide one auditory-visual model or one visual-only stimulus

- Ask the client to produce the sound with a variety of vowels
- Ask the client to produce the sound in both initial and final positions
- Seek 5 productions for each stimulus presentation
- Use a criterion of 80% correct over two sessions or 90% correct in one session

Phase II, Step 2: Word. Goal: Accurate production of target sounds in 25 to 30 varied words to be later included in sentences (nouns, verbs, modifiers, and prepositions).

- Present printed words or picture stimuli
- Ask the client to produce the word
- Accept erred production of nontarget phonemes
- Move training to the sentence level when the sound in a given position (e.g., initial position) is produced with 80% accuracy over two sessions or 90% accuracy in one session
- Continue training at the word level when the sound in a given position (e.g., final position) does not meet the criterion
- Consider using another approach, such as the minimal contrast therapy or phonological process approach, to eliminate the final consonant deletion process

Phase II, Step 3: Phrase and Sentence. Goal: Correct production of all sounds in words; self-monitoring.

- Construct phrases and sentences (imperatives, declaratives, and interrogatives) with words already trained, adding new words as needed
- Present Rebuses, Blissymbolics, or pictures for nonreaders
- Model phrases and sentences
- Ask the client to imitate
- Note phonetic contexts in which errors occur; have the client practice the production in these contexts

- Have the client practice words in which sounds are produced incorrectly as well as those that precede or follow such words
- Vary stress, rhythm, timing, and accent patterns
- Seek 80% accuracy over two sessions or 90% accuracy in one session, calculating accuracy with target sounds only

Phase II. Step 4: Reading and Storytelling. Goal: Accurate production of target sounds in connected utterances containing 4 to 6 words.

- Select reading materials that are easy for the child
- For nonreaders, select comic books, picture books, and sequence cards
- Tell a story and ask the child to retell it
- Seek whole word accuracy and 80 % correct production over two sessions or 90% in one session

Phase II. Step 5: Conversation. Goal: Accurate production of all sounds used in conversational speech.

- Begin to monitor conversational speech when even one or two sounds reach this level
- Encourage discussions, descriptions, comments, questions, state facts, identify cause-effect relations, talk about emotions and desires; not just answer questions
- When multiple sounds need to be monitored, group sounds on the basis of manner or place of articulation; monitor sounds in one group for 3 to 5 minutes; then, monitor sounds in another group, and so on
- Count every spoken word as a response and calculate the whole word accuracy level
- Note the context in which certain sounds are misarticulated and use these contexts for additional practice
- Seek 80% correct production of all words over two sessions or 90% in one session for children 6 years older; seek 69% criterion for younger children

Phase III: Maintenance. Goal: Maintenance of 90% whole word accuracy in conversational speech produced in various speaking situations without treatment or external monitoring.

- Have the client return to the clinic; assess and monitor sound productions
- Visit classrooms
- Maintain telephone contacts with the client and the family
- Obtain report from others
- Have others monitor accuracy in various speaking situations
- Monitor for 3 months

McCabe, R., & Bradley, D. (1975). Systematic multiple phonemic approach to articulation therapy. *Acta Symbolica, 6,* 1–18.

Paired-Stimuli Approach. A method of articulation remediation that depends on identifying a Key Word in which a target sound appears only once in either initial or final position and is correctly produced 9 out of 10 times; uses key words to teach the production of sounds in other contexts; explicitly uses operant reinforcement contingencies; uses pictures to evoke the target words; highly structured and carefully sequenced; a single speech sound is the target at any one time; developed and researched by J. Irwin and A. Weston.

Word Level

Consult Weston and Irwin (1971/1975) for assigned key words, questions to be asked, and expected answers.

- Select the target phonemes for the client
- Find four key words; two containing the target sound in the initial position and two containing it in the final position
- When absent, create key words by teaching them
- Select at least 10 training words in which the target sound is misarticulated and the sound appears only once in the same position as in the key word
- Select pictures as stimuli to evoke the word productions
- Place the **first** key word (picture) with sound in the **initial position** in the center and arrange the 10 training words (pictures) around it

- Point to the key word (picture) and ask the client to, "Say this"
- Reinforce the likely correct production
- Ask the client to name one of the 10 target words
- Ask the child to name the key word again
- Ask the child to name another target word; alternate the key word and a training word in this manner
- Reinforce the client by giving a token for the correct production of the target sound in both the key and the training words; ignore misarticulations of other sounds
- Complete a *training string* by pairing each of the 10 target words with the key word
- Include three training strings in each session that lasts about 30 minutes
- Adhere to a training criterion of 8 correct out of 10 productions of the training words in two successive training strings without reinforcement
- Arrange the **second** key word with the same sound in the **final position** and pair it with 10 training words
- In the next stage of training, ask the child to say the **third** key word with the target sound in the **initial position** and a training word as a Response Unit with only a brief pause between the two (e.g., "said-salad"; *s* is the target; *said* is the key word and *salad* is the target word)
- Reinforce only if the sounds in both the words are correctly produced
- Adhere to a training criterion of 8 out of 10 correct *response units* over two successive training strings
- Ask the child to say the **fourth** key word with the target sound in the **final position** and a training word as a *response unit* with only a brief pause between the two
- Reinforce the correct productions in *response units* as before

Sentence Level

- Pair the **first** key word with its 10 training words; ask a question designed to evoke a response in the sentence form (e.g., "What do you see?" "I *see* a cat" with *see* as the key word for /s/).
- Reinforce with a token on an FR3 schedule of reinforcement
- Complete a training string of 10 questions
- Adhere to the training criterion of 8 out of 10 correct sentences over two training strings
- Alternately, ask two questions (e.g., "What do you see?" for key word *see* and "That's what?" for key word *that's*) as you present the **first** and the **second** key words and their 10 training words
- Reinforce with a token for three correct sentences (FR3)
- Adhere to the training criterion of 8 out of 10 correct sentences over two training strings
- Ask four questions (e.g., "What is this?" "What do you see," "That's what," and "What did you say that was?") as you present the first and the fourth key words and their 10 training words
- Adhere to the criterion of 8 out of 10 correct sentences over two successive training strings

Conversational Level

- Engage the child in conversation
- Stop the conversation (a) when the child correctly produces a target sound in four words or (b) when the child incorrectly produces a target sound in any word; model the correct production; ask the child to repeat it.
- Reinforce the child verbally and by showing your scoring of correct responses
- Subsequently, require the correct production of a target sound in 7 words; probe when the child can do this
- In subsequent stages, require the correct production of a target sound in 10 and 13 words: probe when the child can do this

- Give verbal praise and visual feedback of scoring only when all productions are correct
- For all probes, take a conversational speech sample; no feedback of any sort during probes
- Terminate training on a given sound when the child gives 15 consecutively correct productions of a target sound in conversation held on two successive treatment sessions separated by at least one day

Irwin, J. V., & Weston, A. J. (1971/1975). *Paired Stimuli Kit.* Milwaukee, WI: Fox Point.

Weston, A. J., & Irwin, J. V. (1971). Use of paired stimuli in modification of articulation. *Perceptual Motor Skills, 32,* 947–957.

Phonological Knowledge Approach. An approach to treating phonological disorders in children; based on the assumption that children's knowledge of phonological rules of the adult system is reflected in their productions; the greater the consistency of correct productions in varied contexts, the higher the level of phonological knowledge and vice versa; treatment begins with sounds that reflect least knowledge and ends with those that reflect greater degrees of knowledge; proposed by M. Elbert and J. Gierut and researched by Gierut and associates.

- Obtain a representative, continuous, conversational speech sample
  - sample all sounds
  - sample sounds in all word positions
  - sample each sound in several different words
  - sample each word more than once
  - sample production of minimal pairs (cat/bat)
  - sample morphophonemic alterations (dog/doggie; run/ running)
- Analyze the sample
  - create the child's phonetic inventory (all the sounds the child produces, correctly or incorrectly)
  - create the child's phonemic inventory (sounds the child uses contrastingly or those that signal meaning)

  - find out the distribution of sounds (distribution by word position and by morphemes)
  - create hierarchical arrangement of sound productions that reflect least knowledge (misarticulations in all word positions and in all morphemes) to most knowledge (no misarticulations)
- Treat the sounds that reflect the least knowledge first and move up through the hierarchy
- Use the Contrast Approach (described earlier in this section) in teaching sounds
  - use near-minimal pairs (words that differ by more than one sound) if necessary and initially
  - move from imitation to spontaneous productions
  - reinforce the child for correct productions
  - in spontaneous production training, ask the child to name and sort pictures into target and contrast piles (sorting)
  - present an array of pictures and ask the child to select a picture, name it, and find its minimal pair match (matching)
- Promote generalization and maintenance by varying the context of sound productions, selecting child-specific stimulus items, loosely structuring treatment in later stages, and so forth

Elbert, M., & Gierut, J. (1986). *Handbook of clinical phonology.* San Diego, CA: College-Hill Press.

Phonological Process Approach. An approach to treating articulation disorders; technically, not a treatment procedure; an approach to treatment based on the assumptions that multiple errors reflect the operation of certain phonological rules and that the problem is essentially phonemic, not phonetic; groups errors based on Phonological Processes; targets the elimination of processes; uses several established methods of teaching sounds; researched by multiple investigators.

- Obtain a conversational speech sample that reflects a variety of words and linguistic contexts in which all sounds are produced; may use one of the several available protocols of phonological analysis

- Identify the Phonological Processes that account for error patterns
- Select processes for elimination through teaching specific sounds or groups of sounds
- Teach a few exemplars (sounds) to eliminate a process (e.g., final consonant deletion)
- Probe to see if other, untreated sounds within the pattern are produced correctly without training, based on generalization (e.g., other untreated final consonants that are omitted)
- If there is no generalized production, treat more exemplars
- Schedule maintenance activities as appropriate

Sensory-Motor Approach. An articulation treatment approach based on the assumption that syllable is the basic unit of training; requires a context in which a misarticulated sound is correctly produced; focuses on increasing auditory, tactile, and proprioceptive awareness of motor patterns involved in speech sound production; does not include auditory discrimination training nor training at the sound level; developed and researched by E. McDonald.

- For each target sound find a context in which the child produces it correctly
- If necessary, administer a deep test such as *McDonald's Deep Test of Articulation* to find a context in which an otherwise misarticulated sound is correctly produced (e.g., in the context of *watch-sun*, a child who generally misarticulates the /s/ may produce it correctly)

Practice with sounds produced correctly

- Select a sound the child can produce correctly and combine it with vowels to create duplicated bisyllables (*kiki, koko, kaka, kuku*, etc.)
- Begin treatment by having the child imitate your production of the bisyllables; place equal stress on both the syllables

- Next, have the child imitate your production of bisyllables with primary stress on the first syllable
- Then, have the child imitate your production of bisyllables with primary stress on the second syllable
- Ask the child to describe the placement of the articulators and the direction of the articulatory movements
- Change the vowel and have the child imitate bisyllables with the same consonant but different vowels (e.g., moving from kiki to koko); provide training such that a variety of articulatory movements are practiced for a given sound
- Give similar training with other consonants the child produces correctly
- Initiate training on trisyllables (e.g., kukuku or lalala); follow the procedure used to train bisyllables

Training correct production of misarticulated sounds

Begin training on the typically misarticulated sound with a context in which it is correctly produced (e.g., /s/ is produced correctly in the context of *watch-sun*, a deep test item)

In successive stages, ask the child to say watch-sun:

- with slow motion
- with equal stress on both the syllables
- with primary stress in the first syllable
- with primary stress on the second syllable
- and prolong the /s/ until a signal is given to complete the word
- in sentences ("Watch, the sun will burn you")
- in other and longer sentences and with different stress patterns
- use such a performance criterion as 20 consecutively correct productions to move from one level to the next

Next, vary the phonetic contexts (e.g., watch-sit, watch-saw)

- have the child practice correct production of the target sound in different phonetic contexts by varying the words in which the target sound appears)

- have the child practice correct production in the context of different first words (e.g., *teach-sand, reach-soon*)
- have the child practice the target sound in a totally different phonetic context (e.g., *mop-sun* or *book-sun*)
- implement generalization and maintenance activities

McDonald, E. T. (1964). *Articulation testing and treatment: A sensory motor approach*. Pittsburgh, PA: Stanwix House.

Traditional Approach. An articulation treatment approach developed for the most part by Van Riper who included several techniques from various sources; sounds are trained in isolation, in syllables, in words, and in sentences; training includes four levels: (1) Perceptual Training or Ear Training; (2) Production Training: establishment; (3) production training: stabilizing the productions; and (4) production training: transferring the productions; used or researched by multiple investigators.

Perceptual Training (ear training)

- Demonstrate how the target sound is produced
- Ask the child to raise hand when he or she hears the sound in isolation among sounds that are similar and among sounds that are dissimilar
- Ask the child to raise hand when he or she hears the target sound in first words, then phrases, and finally in sentences
- Ask the child to identify the position of the sound in words (initial, medial, or final)
- Bombard the client with productions of the target sound
- Have the child judge your correct and incorrect productions of a target sound

Production Training

Sound Establishment

- Ask the child to imitate your correct productions of target sounds in isolation, in syllables, or in words
- Vary the phonetic contexts of such productions

- Use contexts in which the target sound is correctly produced
- Use such techniques as Phonetic Placement, Moto-Kinesthetic Method, and Shaping to teach the sound production

Stabilization

- Continue training the **sound in isolation** to encourage more consistent production
- Vary the number and intensity of productions
- Switch from one sound to the other
- Ask the child to respond to printed letters that represent the target sounds
- Have the child produce the sounds in nonsense syllables or clusters
- Begin training the sounds in **words** when the sounds are produced consistently correctly in nonsense syllables
- Move from simple to complex words; continue training until the sound productions are stabilized in a variety of words and in each word position (initial, medial, and final)
- Train at the **phrase** level if necessary
- Move to **sentences**; vary the sentence lengths; move from simpler and shorter to more complex and longer sentences and from those with single occurrence of the target sound to those with multiple occurrences
- Have the child produce sentences along with you in slow motion and at rapid rate
- Begin training at the **conversational level** when the child can fluently and easily produce the target sounds in sentences
- Structure the conversation initially to maximize opportunities for the production of target sounds

- Move to spontaneous conversational speech
- Have the child read to further stabilize sound productions

Transfer (Carry-over)

- Initiate carry-over activities when the child can produce the sounds correctly in unstructured conversational speech
- Give specific speech assignments for the child to complete at home
- Require reports from parents on assignments
- Teach self-monitoring
- Create varied speaking situations for the client to use the target sounds

Van Riper, C. , & Emerick, L. (1984). *Speech correction: An introduction to speech pathology and audiology* (7th ed.). Englewood Cliffs, NJ: Prentice-Hall.

Artificial Larynx. Mechanical larynx used in the communicative rehabilitation of patients with laryngectomy; the same as Electronic Device for Alaryngeal Speech or Pneumatic Device For Alaryngeal Speech.

Assessment. (a) Description and assessment of a client's existing and nonexisting communicative behaviors, background variables, and associated factors to evaluate or diagnose a communicative problem; (b) clinical measurement of a person's communicative behaviors.

- Obtain case history
- Interview client (or caregivers of client)
- Conduct an orofacial examination
- Make client-specific judgments on use of standardized or nonstandardized measures
- Use measures appropriate to the client and his or her cultural background
- Screen hearing
- Obtain a speech-language sample
- Analyze results

- Draw conclusions; make a diagnosis; recommend treatment; disseminate information to the client, the family, and the referring professional

Assimilation Processes. A group of Phonological Processes in which the productions of dissimilar phonemes sound more alike; in phonological treatment, the objective is to eliminate such processes; major assimilation processes include:
- ***Devoicing:*** substitution of a voiceless final sound for a voiced (e.g., /k/ for /g/ in final positions)
- ***Devoicing of final consonants:*** substitution of a voiceless final consonant for a voiced (e.g., /t/ for /d/)
- ***Labial assimilation:*** substitution of a labial sound for a nonlabial (e.g., /b/ for /d/)
- ***Nasal assimilation:*** substitution of a nasal consonant for a non-nasal (e.g., /n/ for /d/)
- ***Prevocalic voicing:*** substitution of a voiced sound for voiceless sound preceding a vowel (e.g., /b/ for /p/ in prevocalic positions)
- ***Reduplication:*** repetition of a syllable, resulting in substitution of one for another (e.g., wawa for *water*)
- ***Velar assimilation:*** substitution of a velar consonant for a nonvelar (e.g., /g/ for /d/)

Assimilative Nasality. Undesirable nasal resonance on vowels that are adjacent to nasal consonants.

Ataxia. A neurological disorder characterized by disturbed balance and movement due to injury to the cerebellum.

Ataxic Dysarthria. A type of motor speech disorder; its neuropathology is damage to the cerebellar system; characterized by slow, inaccurate movement and Hypotonia; all aspects of speech may be involved, but articulatory and prosodic problems dominate; specific symptoms include imprecise consonants, excess and equal linguistic stress, and irregular articulatory breakdowns; select appropriate treatment targets and procedures described under Dysarthria: Treatment; in addition, consider the following that apply especially to ataxic dysarthria:

- Use behavioral methods of Shaping and Differential Reinforcement to improve control and coordination
- Reinforce slower speech rate to improve intelligibility
- Modify prosody, including excess loudness variation
- Reinforce more natural sounding speech
- Do not concentrate on increasing muscle strength or reducing muscle tone
- Do not recommend prosthetic or surgical methods to improve phonation or resonance

Duffy, J. R. (1995). *Motor speech disorders.* St. Louis, MO: C. V. Mosby.

Johns, D. F. (Ed.). (1985). *Clinical management of neurogenic communicative disorders*. Boston: Little, Brown

Yorkston, K. M., Beukelman, D. R., & Bell, K. R. (1988). *Clinical management of dysarthric speakers.* Austin, TX: Pro-Ed.

Athetosis. A neurological disorder characterized by slow, writhing, worm-like movements due to injury to the extrapyramidal motor pathways.

Atrophy. Wasting away of tissues or organs.

Audience Generalization. Production of unreinforced responses in the presence of persons not involved in training.

- Evoke behavior
- Reinforce target behavior

Auditory Discrimination Training. Treatment designed to teach clients to distinguish between correct and incorrect productions of speech sounds; used on the assumption that auditory discrimination training is a precursor to speech sound production training; assumption questioned by some clinicians who believe that production training will induce discrimination as well; same as Perceptual Training.

Augmentative Communication. Methods of communication that enhance and expand extremely limited oral means of communication by nonvocal means; some augmentative communication may involve speech generated mechanically; includes various means of communication some of which are more technologically oriented than others; usually used for persons who have limited oral communication skills because of severe clinical conditions including aphasia, autism, cerebral palsy, and other neurological disorders, deafness, dementia, dysarthria, glossectomy, intubation, laryngectomy, mental retardation, tracheostomy, and traumatic head injury; for procedures, see Augmentative Communication, Gestural (Unaided); Augmentative Communication, Gestural-Assisted (Aided); Augmentative Communication, Neuro-Assisted (Aided).

Basic principles of selecting an augmentative communication mode or system

- Assess the client's speech as well as nonspeech communication potential
- Consider the client's strengths and limitations
  - cognitive level
  - sensory disabilities
  - motor status
  - language comprehension
- Select a mode or system that gives the maximum advantage to the client
- Consider cost
- Consider the client's acceptance of the mode or system
- Consider the communicative demands the client faces
- Consider the amount of training required
- Consider how the client and the family will use the mode or system

Augmentative Communication, Aided. Methods of communication that enhance or expand (and rarely substitute) vocal communication by such external aids as an alphabet letter board or a computer.

Augmentative Communication, Gestural (unaided). Methods of communication that use patterned muscle movements (gestures) to enhance oral communication but do not use instruments or external aids; gestures play a crucial role in conveying the speaker's message; appropriate for all persons with severely impaired oral, expressive communication.

- Teach gestures for *Yes* and *No* to all speakers with extremely limited expressive oral communication because of severely impaired motor performance but relatively intact receptive language
  - teach the client to gesture *Yes* or *No* in response to a series of common questions with a carrier phrase "Do you want _____?"
  - shape a clear gesture that all communication partners can understand
  - model the gesture if necessary
  - reinforce consistently discriminated responding (client always gives the gesture that is meant)
  - consider the following gestures: head movements (side to side for *No* and up and down for *Yes*); eye movements (looking up for *Yes* and down for *No*; blinking once for *Yes* and twice for *No*; blinking the right eye for *Yes* and the left eye for *No*); hand movements (thumbs up for *Yes* and thumbs down for *No*;) feet movements (right foot movement for *Yes* and the left foot movement for *No*)
- Teach a pattern of eye-blinks that convey certain basic messages; for instance, beyond the *Yes* and *No* teach the client to:
  - blink three times to say *I am hungry*
  - four times to say *I am thirsty*
  - five times to say *I need to go to bathroom*
- Teach pointing to objects needed
  - teach finger pointing
  - teach pointing by directing gaze
- Teach the Left-Hand Manual Alphabet
  - consider teaching the left-hand manual alphabet for clients whose right hand is paralyzed
  - consider teaching the Manual Shorthand which combines gestures with letters from the left-hand manual alphabet *(talking hand system)*

- Teach Pantomime
  - teach the client to use pantomime along with speech
  - teach initially a few mimed concepts that help communicate basic needs
  - expand the mimed repertoire as the client becomes more competent in its use
  - fade mimes if and when the client regains or improves oral speech
- Teach American Indian Hand Talk (AMER-IND)
  - teach first the signs that express mands (basic needs, requests)
  - teach the one-hand version for those with one paralyzed hand
  - teach signs that express concrete ideas first and those that express abstract ideas later
- Teach American Sign Language (ASL or AMESLAN)
  - select initially the signs that express Mands (basic needs, requests)
  - teach signs that express concrete ideas first and those that express abstract ideas later

Beukelman, D. R., & Mirenda, P. (1992). *Augmentative and alternative communication: Management of severe communication disorders in children and adults.* Baltimore, MD: Paul H. Brooks.

Silverman, F. H. (1995). *Communication for the speechless* (3rd ed.). Boston: Allyn & Bacon.

Augmentative Communication, Gestural-assisted (aided). Methods of communication in which gestures are used to (a) select or scan messages displayed on a nonmechanical device (e.g., a communication board) or (b) display messages on a mechanical device (e.g., a computer monitor); used with many persons with minimal expressive language; the initial use of gestural-assisted means may promote appropriate vocalization or word productions in many clients; the emergent vocal productions may be strengthened and expanded; includes a variety of nonmechanical and mechanical methods.

Use pictures and symbols to teach functional communication

- Teach the client to communicate with photographs and drawings that may be displayed on a communication board
  - teach the client with limited cognitive functions to communicate basic needs with regular or miniaturized objects (e.g., the client points to a fork to indicate he or she wants to eat)
  - teach the client to express a particular message through a picture (e.g., teach the client to point to or look at a picture of a person sleeping to communicate that he or she is tired or sleepy)
  - teach the client to express bodily states (e.g., pain in a certain part) by pointing to or looking at specific body parts on a line drawing
- Teach the client to communicate with various symbols that may be displayed on a communication board; select among many symbol systems that are available on the market:
  - Picsyms, a set of graphic symbols that represent nouns, verbs, and prepositions
  - Pic Symbols (Pictogram Ideogram Communication) which are white drawings on a black background
  - Sig symbols which are based on *American Sign Language (ASL)*; use them especially in conjunction with ASL
  - Blissymbolics which are a set of semi-iconic and abstract symbols that can be taught to persons of any language; teach the client to combine symbols to form more complex messages
  - Premack-type Symbols, or the Carrier Symbols which are abstract plastic shapes; associate words and phrases with each shape; teach the client to arrange and rearrange the plastic shapes like printed words
  - traditional orthography (e.g., the English alphabet); teach the client to spell out the word (by pointing to or scanning) along with the alphabet, display digits 1 through 10 and a set of common phrases or sentences so that not

every word has to be spelled out or scanned (Scanning in Augmentative Communication)

- Teach the client to communicate with Rebuses
  - use rebuses (pictures that represent objects or events along with words, grammatic morphemes, or both)
  - teach the client to add grammatic morphemes to a picture or a word (e.g., adding s to the picture of a book to suggest *books*)
  - combine rebuses to form more complex utterances

Use nonelectronic communication boards to teach functional communication

- Teach the client to communicate with messages on a nonelectronic communication board
  - design a board of paper, cardboard, fabric, wood, or cork; if practical, prepare a book of symbols and written messages; select a board that all conversational partners can see simultaneously; portable, if necessary; attractive to look at; big enough to contain critical elements of the system; not overwhelmingly big or complex
  - write symbols (alphabets, orthographic messages, pictures, various kinds of symbols) on separate cards that can be mounted on the board
  - teach the client who cannot point (because of extremely limited motoric performance) to scan the message: you offer selections and the client indicates yes to the right selection (e.g., you point to the word "food," or a symbol for it, or a picture of a food item; the client indicates *Yes* or *No*)
  - teach the client to encode a message by pointing to a number printed on a separate, smaller, portable selection chart; have the messages on a larger communication board numbered: let the client point to a number on the selection chart; decode the number into the message on the board (e.g., if the client points to #5, it may mean "I am hungry" as per the communication board)
  - teach the client to directly select the message: teach the client to select the actual message on the board, instead

of a number which stands for a message; teach clients to select by means of pointing and other hand gestures, finger movements, eye gestures, gaze, headpointers, or headsticks.

- Teach the client to communicate by drawing symbols or pictures
  - teach the client to draw simple line drawings to communicate
  - let the client use paper, magic slate, or any other convenient surface
- Teach the client to communicate by writing (Traditional Orthography)
  - teach conventional writing to nonverbal children who can master it
  - teach them initially to write simple, functional messages
  - teach them to write more complex messages

Use electronic communication systems to teach functional communication

- Select an appropriate system for the client; consider the cost, ease of use, and efficiency of the system
- Select an appropriate and practical switching mechanism that the client can use with little effort and learning to generate signals for the electronic device (such as those that are specially constructed or a modified or regular microcomputer); consider push switches, push plates (plate-like structures that when touched will generate a signal) large and specially designed keyboards, joy sticks, squeeze bulbs, and several other available types of selection devices
- Select an appropriate display system to show messages when the client activates the switching mechanism; these may be computer screens, liquid-crystal displays (found on calculators), printed outputs (as with a computer printer), and many other kinds of special displays
- Select an appropriate control electronic unit (a dedicated augmentative communication unit or a computer)
- Teach the client in using the device; start with simpler messages; give plenty of practice in using the switching mech-

anism; increase the complexity of messages in gradual steps; train the communicative partners in the environment

Beukelman, D. R., & Mirenda, P. (1992). *Augmentative and alternative communication: Management of severe communication disorders in children and adults*. Baltimore, MD: Paul H. Brooks.

Silverman, F. H. (1995). *Communication for the speechless* (3rd ed.). Boston: Allyn and Bacon.

Augmentative Communication, High Technology. Methods of communication that enhance or expand (and rarely substitute for) vocal communication by external means that use sophisticated electronic technology, including computers; generate speech or printed messages; usually software run; more versatile than low-technology augmentative communication.

Augmentative Communication, Low Technology. Methods of communication that enhance or expand (and rarely substitute) vocal communication by external means that use no or limited electronic technology; there is no message storage, printed output, or speech output; a communication board with letters and words on it is an example.

Augmentative Communication, Neuro-assisted (aided). Methods of communication that use such bioelectrical signals as muscle action potentials to activate and display messages on a computer monitor; technically, a variety of switching device; used for persons who are so profoundly impaired motorically that they cannot use a manual switching device; the communicator needs to have electrodes attached to the skin surface to pickup and transmit muscle action potential signals to the device; this technology not well developed.

- Train the client to use muscle action potentials to generate signals to an electronic communication device
  - teach the client to vary muscle action potentials through biofeedback training
  - use a myoswitch that picks up muscle action potential from contracting muscles and transmits the impulse to an electronic device

use any of the several electronic devices available that have been modified for this purpose

Beukelman, D. R., & Mirenda, P. (1992). *Augmentative and alternative communication: Management of severe communication disorders in children and adults.* Baltimore, MD: Paul H. Brooks.

Silverman, F. H. (1995). *Communication for the speechless* (3rd ed.). Boston: Allyn & Bacon.

Augmentative Communication, Unaided. Methods of communication that enhance or expand (and rarely substitute for) vocal communication without external or mechanical aids; includes a more formal, systematic, intensive, or extensive use of gestures, signs, and facial expressions to supplement oral (speech) communication.

Aural Rehabilitation. An educational and clinical program implemented, for the most part, by audiologists; includes the assessment of hearing impairment in adults and children; counseling; selection and fitting of hearing aids and auditory training; use of group amplification systems in educational and communication training sessions; often implemented by a team of specialists including audiologist, otologist, special education specialists, psychologists, and speech-language pathologists; see Hard of Hearing; Hearing Impairment; and Hearing Loss.

Autism: A pervasive developmental disorder that in a majority of clients persists into adulthood; often associated with mental retardation; communication disorders are a significant characteristic; lack of interest in people and communication is a dominant characteristic; many of the treatment procedures for Language Disorders in Children are applicable with the following special considerations:

- Use objects, not pictures, as stimuli
- Teach in a variety of linguistic contexts
- Teach in a variety of environments
- Reduce Echolalia
- Give direct, intensive training

- Pay special attention to generalization and maintenance strategies
- Teach nonverbal communication (e.g., American Sign Language) if necessary
- Work closely with other specialists and family members

Automatic Reinforcers. Sensory consequences of responses that reinforce those responses (e.g., the sensation a child with autism derives from banging his or her head).

Autosomal Dominant. Any chromosome apart from the sex chromosome is autosomal; not sex-linked; dominant indicates that the defective gene dominates its normal partner in its phenotypic expression.

Aversive Stimuli. Events that people work hard to avoid or move away from; reduction in aversive stimulation is the essence of negative reinforcement; a behavior that reduces negative experiences tends to increase in frequency; in treatment, positive reinforcement is preferable to negative reinforcement.

Avoidance. A behavior that prevents the occurrence of an aversive event and hence is reinforced; negatively reinforced behavior; in treatment, target is to reduce avoidance if judged undesirable; for instance, in reducing avoidance of certain speaking situations by persons who stutter:
- Build a hierarchy of most to least frequently avoided speaking situations or tasks
- As the client becomes more fluent during treatment, introduce the client to least frequently avoided situations first and move up the hierarchy
- Reinforce the client for facing previously avoided situations and tasks

Backup Reinforcers. Events, objects, and opportunities for selected behaviors that become available to clients who exchange their earned tokens in treatment sessions.

- Have a collection of back-up reinforcers
- Give tokens to reinforce target responses
- Exchange tokens for selected events, objects, or opportunities for certain behaviors

Basal Ganglia. Structures located deep within the brain and just above midbrain that are important for movement control; part of the extrapyramidal system; include the caudate nucleus, the putamen nucleus, and globus pallidus.

Baselines. Recorded rates of responses in the absence of planned intervention; reliability or stability of repeated measures is a required characteristic; help establish the clinician accountability; in treatment research, help rule out extraneous variables.

- Specify target behaviors
- Prepare stimulus items to evoke target responses
- Use objects, modeling, questions
- Prepare recording sheet
- Administer baseline trials
- Select type: Baseline Evoked Trials or Baseline Modeled Trials
- Analyze data to calculate percentage of correct responses
- Repeat measures
- When measures are stable, begin treatment

Baseline Evoked Trials. Discrete baseline trials that are temporally separated; each attempt to produce a target behavior is discretely measured; no modeling of the target response; no consequences for the correct or incorrect responses.

- Place stimulus item in front of the client or demonstrate an action
- Ask the relevant predetermined question
- Wait a few seconds for the client to respond

- Record the client's response on the recording sheet
- Remove stimulus item
- Wait 2–3 seconds to signify end of trial

Baseline Modeled Trials. A discrete baseline trial in which the clinician models the correct response for the client to imitate; no consequences for the correct or incorrect responses.
- Place a stimulus item in front of client or demonstrate an action
- Ask the predetermined question
- Immediately model the correct response
- Wait a few seconds for the client to respond
- Record the client's response on the recording sheet
- Remove the stimulus item
- Wait 2–3 seconds to signify end of trial

Behavioral Contingency. In behavioral analysis and treatment, a dependent relationship between Antecedents, responses, and Consequences; in behavioral treatment, clinician manages this contingency by:
- Providing antecedents (stimuli, modeling, instruction, demonstration, etc.)
- Requiring a specified response
- Providing immediate consequences in the form of positive reinforcers or corrective feedback

Behavioral Momentum. A behavioral treatment procedure in which the clinician rapidly and repeatedly evokes a high-probability response and then immediately commands a low-probability response; often used to reduce noncompliance; in increasing the frequency of a low-probability response:
- Find a response the client readily performs (e.g., hand clapping)
- Model and have the child imitate that high-probability response repeatedly and in rapid succession
- Immediately, ask the child to open his or her mouth (an example of a low- probability response)
- Reinforce the occurrence of the low probability response

Biofeedback. A method used to reduce incorrect responses or shape and increase desirable responses in treatment; includes mechanical feedback given to the client on vocal pitch and intensity, respiration, galvanic skin response, and muscle action potential level.

Bite Block. A small block of acrylic or putty custom-made for a client who holds it between the lateral upper and lower teeth; observed to improve speech intelligibility in clients who have abnormal jaw movements; recommended for some clients with dysarthria.

Blissymbolics. A set of symbols used to communicate nonorally; meant to be an international language; more widely applied and researched than other symbol systems in teaching communication to severely handicapped clients; symbols may be combined to form complex expressions; Developed by C. Bliss; see Augmentative Communication, Gestural-Assisted (Aided).

Bolus. A mass of chewed or otherwise prepared food moved as a unit in the act of swallowing.

Booster Treatment. Treatment given any time after the client was dismissed from the original treatment; part of response maintenance strategy.

- Conduct periodic follow-ups
- If the follow-up measures show decline in response rate, give booster treatment
- Use the original or newer, more effective procedures

Botulinum Toxin Injection. A medical treatment procedure for neurogenic or idiopathic adductor spasmodic dysphonia and adductor spasmodic dysphonia that does not respond to behavioral treatment; botulinum toxin is injected into the thyroarytenoid muscle unilaterally or bilaterally; effects last about 3 months.

Bradykinesia. Slowness of movements; difficulty in stopping movement once initiated; freezing of movement.

Breathiness. A voice quality that results when there is excessive air leakage during phonation because of inadequate approximation of the vocal folds; caused by various factors; treatment varies by cause.

Carrier Symbols. A set of plastic symbols (adapted from the Premack symbols) used in teaching nonverbal communication; used as a part of the Non-SLIP (Non-Speech Language Initiation Program); once learned, the program helps initiate oral speech training; developed and researched by J. Carrier.

Carry-over. Generalized production of any behavior taught in a special setting in natural and untreated settings and in relation to novel stimuli; an important goal of clinical intervention; the same as Generalization.

Cerebral Palsy. A congenital, nonprogressive neurological disorder that affects motor control; caused by injury to the cerebral levels during the prenatal or perinatal period; symptoms tend to improve with growth; causes speech disorders, mostly dysarthria; symptoms related to speech include respiratory control problems, laryngeal dysfunction resulting in voice problems, possible velopharyngeal inadequacy, potential language disorders, and significant articulation problems (dysarthria); may involve cognitive functions; may be associated with feeding problems.

Classification of Cerebral Palsy

- *Ataxic Cerebral Palsy*: Ataxia, disturbed balance and movement, is the main characteristic; injury to the cerebellum.
- *Athetoid Cerebral Palsy*: Athetosis, characterized by slow, involuntary, writhing movements, is the distinguishing feature; injury to the extrapyramidal motor pathways, especially to the basal ganglia.
- *Spastic Cerebral Palsy*: Increased tone or rigidity of muscles is the distinguishing feature; the most common type; injury to the pyramidal motor pathways and the higher cortical centers of motor control.

Treatment of Cerebral Palsy

General Principles

- Work closely with the team of specialists serving children with cerebral palsy
- Counsel parents about the effects of cerebral palsy on communication and their role in stimulating language at home

- Work closely with parents throughout the treatment duration
- Make a thorough assessment of communication problems and design treatment to suit the child's problems, needs, and strengths
- Consider educational demands made or to be made on the child in planning treatment; work closely with educators
- Borrow techniques from other communicative disorders in children (e.g., language disorders, articulation and phonological disorders, dysarthria, voice disorders) as cerebral palsy is not the name of a unique speech disorder; modify the standard techniques to suit the individual child and his or her specific symptom complex

Treatment Procedures

- Treatment of language disorders

  train parents to stimulate language at home; see Parent Training and Language Stimulation by Parents

  assess the child's language development periodically to determine the need for formal clinical treatment

  implement formal language treatment if necessary

  use the treatment procedures described under Language Disorders in Children and modify the procedures to suit the individual child with cerebral palsy
- Treatment of voice disorders
  - diagnose the specific voice disorder; when appropriate, use one or more treatment techniques described under Voice Disorders with suitable modifications; be aware that voice disorders may be due to respiratory problems associated with cerebral palsy
  - treat associated respiratory problems; prescribe exercises to improve breath support for speech; use techniques described under Dysarthria, Treatment
  - treat velopharyngeal incompetence only if there is enough tissue mass and behavioral training thus is likely to be effective; see Treatment of Voice Disorders and Treatment of Disorders of Resonance

- Treatment of articulation and phonological disorders
  - assess the child's specific sound errors and error patterns
  - assess the compensatory articulatory postures the child uses
  - modify or eliminate inappropriate and ineffective compensatory postures
  - teach the specific phonemes or classes of phonemes based on distinctive features or phonological patterns
  - use the treatment techniques described under Articulation and Phonological Disorders with appropriate modifications

Changing Criterion, Research Design. A single-subject research design to evaluate treatment effects; effectiveness of a treatment is demonstrated by effecting changes in target behaviors that approximate a changing criterion of performance; in successive stages of treatment, the behavior is held to a lower or higher criterion.

Changing Criterion, Treatment Procedure. A method of shaping desirable behaviors by using performance criteria that change every time the client meets a certain criterion; the criterion may change in either direction (lower or higher) depending on the target behavior; in reducing the speech rate of clients with certain communicative disorders, the criteria are progressively lower; in shaping longer utterances, the criteria are progressively higher.

Chant-Talk. A voice therapy technique characterized by speech that resembles chanting; consists of soft glottal attacks; raised pitch, prolonged syllables, even stress, and smooth blending of words; considered appropriate for hyperfunctional voice problems; helps reduce excessive muscular effort and tension associated with voice production; for procedures, See Specific Normal Voice Facilitating Techniques under Voice Disorders.

Chewing Method. A voice therapy technique used to reduce vocal hyperfunction; helps reduce excessive tension and muscular effort associated with voice production; for procedures, see Specific Normal Voice Facilitating Techniques under Voice Disorders.

Child-Centered Approach. A child language intervention approach which assigns a more active role to the child; play-oriented and indirect treatment method; clinician takes the child's lead in targeting language structures for intervention; see Language Disorders in Children; Treatment of Language Disorders: Specific Techniques or Programs.

Childhood Aphasia (Congenital Aphasia). A controversial and somewhat dated term used to describe certain children's language disorders that could not be explained on the basis of other known variables including neurological problems, hearing impairment, mental retardation, environmental deficit, and so forth; a diagnosis made on negative evidence; questioned or rejected by many clinicians.

Choreiform Movements. Jerky, irregular, involuntary, and rapid movements; caused by damage to the caudate and the putamen; major symptom of Huntington's Disease.

Circumlocutions. Talking around a theme or failing to use specific terms.

Cleft. An opening in a structure that is normally closed.

Cleft Lip. Opening in the upper lip; may be on one (unilateral) or both (bilateral) the sides of the lip; due to failure in embryonic growth processes.

Cleft Palate. Opening in the palate, the structure that separates the oral and nasal cavities; varies in extent and severity and may extend from the upper lip to the soft palate; due to failures in embryonic growth processes.

Surgical Management of the Clefts

- *Lip surgery*. Surgical methods to close unilateral or bilateral clefts; usually done when the baby is about 3 months old or weighs about 10 pounds.

- *Palatal surgery*. Surgical procedures performed to close the cleft or clefts of the palate; done when the baby is between 9 and 24 months, many between 9 and 12 months; the earlier the closure of the cleft, the better the speech development.
- *V-Y Retroposition*. A surgical method to repair the cleft of the palate; also known as Veau-Wardill-Kilner procedure; clefts are closed by raising from the bone single-based flaps of palatal mucoperiosteum on either side of the cleft and closing the cleft with the flaps as they are pushed back to lengthen the palate; improves chances of better speech production.
- *von Langenbeck Method*. A surgical method to repair the cleft of the palate by raising two bipedicled (attached on both ends) flaps of mucoperiosteum, bringing them together, and attaching them; leaves denuded bone on either side; does not lengthen the palate.
- *Delayed Hard Palate Closure*. A surgical sequence to close the cleft in which the soft palatal cleft is closed first and the hard palatal cleft is closed later.
- *Primary Surgery for the Clefts*. The initial surgery in which the clefts are closed.
- *Pharyngeal Flap*. A secondary palatal surgical procedure designed to improve the velopharyngeal functioning for speech; a muscular flap is cut from the posterior pharyngeal wall, raised, and attached to the velum; the flap is open on either side to allow for nasal breathing, nasal drainage, and production of nasal speech sounds; helps close the velopharyngeal port and thus reduce hypernasality.
- *Pharyngoplasty*. A surgical procedure designed to improve velopharyngeal incompetence; such substances as Teflon®, silicone, dacron wool/silicone gel bag, and cartilage may be implanted or injected into the posterior pharyngeal wall to make it bulge and thus help close the velopharyngeal port.
- *Secondary surgeries for clefts*. Surgical procedures done after the primary surgery to improve functioning and appearance.

McWilliams, B. J., Morris, H. L., & Shelton, R. L. (1990). *Cleft palate speech* (2nd ed.). Philadelphia: B. C. Decker.

Cleft Lip and Palate: Treatment for Articulation and Phonological Disorders

General Principles

- A thorough assessment of articulation skills and velopharyngeal function is necessary before starting treatment
- Treatment is effective if the child has at least a marginal velopharyngeal competence
- Children with significant velopharyngeal incompetence need surgery, prosthetic assistance, or both
- Treatment should be offered as early as possible
- Treatment should emphasize production and not auditory discrimination
- Trial therapy may be needed to determine prognosis
- Behavioral principles and procedures are effective in teaching correct articulation
- Phonological approach may be appropriate in certain children with repaired cleft
- Many techniques used to treat Articulation and Phonological Disorders in children without clefts are appropriate in teaching sound production to children with repaired clefts

Treatment Procedures: Articulation and Phonological Disorders

Use the procedures of treating Articulation and Phonological Disorders; consider the following suggestions, some of which are unique to children with repaired clefts.

- Educate parents about the speech mechanism
- Withhold reinforcement for undesirable compensatory behaviors the need for which has been eliminated by medical treatment
- Teach the more visible sounds before the less visible except for the linguadentals
- Teach stops and fricatives before other class of sounds

- Avoid or postpone training on /k/ and /g/ if the velopharyngeal functioning is inadequate
- Teach fricatives, affricates, or both if they are stimulable or after stops are mastered
- Teach linguapalatal sounds, lingualveolars, and linguadentals in that order
- Progress from syllables to words, phrases, and sentences
- Give auditory and visual cues; model frequently
- Provide systematic practice and reinforce correct productions
- Introduce compensatory articulatory positioning where appropriate
- Teach the client to direct the breath stream orally; let the child feel the airstream on hand or see the movement of a piece of tissue
- Teach the child to avoid posterior articulatory placements
- Teach the child to articulate with less effort and facial grimacing
- Give tactile cues and instruction to improve tongue positioning
- Work on generalization and maintenance; train parents to reinforce correct articulation at home

McWilliams, B. J., Morris, H. L., & Shelton, R. L. (1990). *Cleft palate speech* (2nd ed.). Philadelphia: B. C. Decker.

Cleft Lip and Palate: Treatment of Language Disorders

General Principles

- Language stimulation by parents may be all that is needed in some cases
- Formal language treatment may be necessary in some cases
- Need to work with the parents from early infancy to establish a long-term rapport
- Counseling parents about language development is essential

- The basic language treatment procedures are not much different from those used with Language Disorders in Children without clefts

Treatment Procedures: Language Disorders

Use the procedures of treating Language Disorders in Children without clefts; consider the following suggestions, some of which are unique to children with clefts:

- Teach parents to stimulate language at home
- Ask parents to encourage free verbal expression in their child
- Ask parents to integrate stimulation for articulation and language
- Integrate information about all aspects of rehabilitation in your discussion with the parents
- Ask parents to socially reinforce the child's spontaneous verbal productions
- Teach parents to reduce negative feedback, and make more positive statements about the child's communicative attempts
- Meet with parents regularly to review progress and modify their home language stimulation program
- Periodically assess the child's language skills
- Start formal language treatment when one of the periodic assessments warrant it
- Consider the imminent educational demands and plan language intervention to help meet them

Cleft Lip and Palate: Treatment of Phonatory Disorders

General Principles

- Phonatory problems may be due to compensatory behaviors or may be independent of velopharyngeal insufficiency
- Use techniques described under Voice Disorders if the problems are independent of velopharyngeal insufficiency (and due to vocal abuse)

- Consider phonatory treatment as diagnostic; discontinue if there is no improvement in phonatory problems or other speech symptoms worsen
- Do not try to eliminate nasal escape and hypernasality
- Do not offer phonatory treatment for children with a clear diagnosis of velopharyngeal incompetence
- Follow treated children because some improve, some deteriorate, and some stay the same

Treatment Procedures for Hyperfunctional Voice

- Describe how voice is produced to the child and the parents
- Reduce Vocally Abusive Behaviors in the child and in other members of the family
- Counsel the family about good vocal behaviors (e.g., talking less in noisy environments, practicing soft speech, good conversational turn taking, clapping instead of shouting or yelling)
- Use auditory discrimination training by helping the child to discriminate his or her voice from that of other children without vocal nodules or other vocal pathology
- Use such biofeedback instruments as the Visi-Pitch™ in training
- Train healthy voice production by teaching the child to
  - reduce vocal loudness
  - eliminate hard glottal attacks
  - initiate words that start with vowels
  - use easy, gentle onset of phonation
  - self-monitor voice

McWilliams, B. J., Morris, H. L., & Shelton, R. L. (1990). *Cleft palate speech* (2nd. ed.). Philadelphia: B. C. Decker.

Cleft Lip and Palate: Treatment for Resonance Disorders

General Principles

- Do not treat *Hypernasality* if it is a result of velopharyngeal incompetence
- Treat hypernasality only if the child is capable of achieving velopharyngeal closure

- See if surgery reduces or eliminates hypernasality; improvement may continue for up to a year following surgery

Treatment Procedures: Resonance Disorders

- Use techniques described under <u>Voice Disorders</u> to reduce hypernasality including increased loudness, discrimination training to distinguish oral and nasal resonance, lowered pitch, and increased oral opening
- Use respiratory training to improve loudness
- Attempt articulation with the nares occluded
- Decrease intra-oral breath pressure on stop consonants and fricatives, while simultaneously using loose articulatory contacts
- Use such biofeedback instruments as Tonar II™ to reduce hypernasality
- Use the whistle-blowing technique of R. M. Shprintzen and his associates to promote velopharyngeal closure during speech
  - teach whistling and blowing at the same time
  - reinforce when nasal airflow is absent
  - continue until there is no nasal escape during whistling or blowing
  - eliminate whistling or blowing, and introduce phonation
  - continue until no nasal escape is evident
  - introduce vowels /i/ or /u/ while blowing or whistling
  - continue until there is no longer nasal escape
  - eliminate blowing or whistling, and produce only the vowels
  - form monosyllables by using non-nasal consonants with vowels
  - move to words, sentences, and conversations
  - teach self-monitoring skills

Boone, D. R., & McFarlane, S. C. (1988). *The voice and voice therapy* (4th ed). Englewood Cliffs, NJ: Prentice-Hall.

McWilliams, B. J., Morris, H. L., & Shelton, R. L. (1990). *Cleft palate speech* (2nd. ed.). Philadelphia: B. C. Decker.

Wilson, D. K. (1972). *Voice problems in children*. Baltimore, MD: Williams & Wilkins.

Client-specific Strategy. A method of selecting target behaviors that are relevant and useful for the individual client.

Observe client's environment for clues
Select useful and relevant target behaviors
Consider potential for generalization
Must serve as building blocks for new behaviors

Closed-Head Injury. The same as <u>Nonpenetrating Head Injury</u>.

Cloze Procedure. Modeling parts of an utterance and pausing for the child to produce words and phrases to complete the utterance; the same as <u>Partial Modeling</u> and <u>Completion</u>.

- Model only the initial portion of a target response (e.g., say "The boy is. . ." and wait for the response)
- Let the child complete the partial model (e.g., the child says "walking")
- Reinforce the child's response

Cluttering. A speech-language disorder characterized by rapid speech rate, irregular speech rate, or both; a fluency disorder related to, but different from, stuttering; may co-exist with stuttering; also defined as a fluency disorder with rapid rate, indistinct articulation, and impaired language formulation possibly suggesting poor organization of thought with reduced or absent awareness or concern about the problems; certain elements of treatment are common to stuttering and cluttering.

General Guidelines

- Make a thorough assessment of the overall symptoms; determine the extent of fluency, articulation, and language problems
- Teach a slower rate of speech
- Teach syllable prolongation
- Use <u>Metronome-Paced Speech</u> or <u>Delayed Auditory Feedback (both described under Stuttering; Treatment of Stuttering: Specific Techniques or Programs)</u> if necessary to slow the rate and induce prolongation

- Use Shadowing (described under Stuttering; Treatment of Stuttering: Specific Techniques or Programs)
- Teach slow and distinct articulation
- Teach pausing between clauses and sentences
- Ask the client to increase the rate beyond baseline and then slow down to encourage discrimination
- Correct any phoneme-specific misarticulations through methods of treating Articulation and Phonological Disorders
- Teach the client to produce syllables with deliberate stress, especially the final and unstressed syllables of words
- Tape record the client's cluttered speech and play it back to increase awareness
- Give prompt, contingent feedback on cluttered speech to increase awareness
- Heighten clutterers' awareness of their listeners' difficulty in understanding them; sensitize the clients to the listener's facial expressions and gestures that signal difficulty in understanding
- Treat word finding difficulties by having the client name rapidly and learn words in semantically varied categories
- Teach conversational turn taking, organized expressions, and coherent talking
- Teach Self-Control (Self-Monitoring) Skills
- Implement a maintenance program
- Follow-up and give booster treatment

Myers, F. L., & St. Louis, K. O. (1992). *Cluttering: A clinical perspective.* Kibworth, England: Far Communications.

Rate Reduction in Treating Cluttering

A speech rate slower than the normal or below a client-specific baserate; a typical target to improve speech intelligibility and to reduce dysfluencies of persons who clutter; may use Delayed Auditory Feedback (DAF) to induce rate reduction.

- Establish a baserate of speech rate measured either in syllables or words per minute
- Instruct the client in rate reduction and describe its desirable effects

- Reassure the client that a more acceptable rate is the final target of treatment
- Model a slow rate of speech for the client
- Model pausing at appropriate junctures
- Experiment with slower rates and increased frequency or duration of pauses that result in reduced or eliminated dysfluencies and improved intelligibility
- Model the effective rate selected for the client
- Ask the client to imitate the reduced rate
- Use delayed auditory feedback if instructions and modeling are not effective
- Start with words and phrases and move on to controlled and spontaneous sentences
- Add other targets (distinct articulation, increased stress, prolonged vowels)
- Fade excessively slow rate while maintaining distinct articulation and decreased dysfluencies
- Teach self-monitoring skills
- Follow-up and arrange for booster treatment

Collaborative Model. A service delivery model used in public schools; the speech-language pathologist works with the classroom teacher in identifying clinical activities that promote academic learning in a child with communication disorders; the clinician works in the classroom along with the teacher.

Collagen Injection. A medical treatment procedure for clients with paralyzed vocal cords; injected into the middle third of the cord, collagen increases the bulk and the chances of abduction.

Completion. The same as Cloze Procedure and Partial Modeling.

Conditioned Generalized Reinforcers. Tokens, money, and other reinforcers that are effective in a wide range of conditions; Secondary Reinforcers that have a generalized effect; use them to:

- Promote generalized productions of target behaviors
- Enhance the effectiveness of reinforcers used in treatment

Conditioned Reinforcers. events that reinforce behaviors because of past learning experiences; the same as Secondary Reinforcers.

Concurrent Stimulus-Response Generalization. Production of new and unreinforced responses in relation to new stimuli; the most complex form of generalized production.

Confrontation Naming. Naming a stimulus when asked to do so; a correct response to such questions as "What is this?"

Congenital Aphasia. The same as Childhood Aphasia.

Congenital Palatopharyngeal Incompetence. An inadequate velopharyngeal mechanism that cannot close the velopharyngeal port for the production of non-nasal speech sounds; not due to clefts; hard palate may be too short or the nasopharynx may be too deep; speech is hypernasal; depending on the degree of incompetence, resonance (voice) therapy may be ineffective without surgical or prosthetic help.

Consequences. Events that follow a response and thus increase or decrease the future probability of those responses; in treatment, clinician's differential response to client's correct, incorrect, and no response.

Constituent Definitions. Dictionary definitions of terms with no reference to how what is defined is measured (e.g., *the goal of treatment is to reduce stuttering*) contrasted with Operational Definitions (e.g., *the goal of treatment is to reduce specified dysfluencies to below 3% of the words spoken*).

Consultant Model. A service delivery model; the speech-language pathologist selects the training targets and procedures; trains teachers, parents, siblings, aides, and others who actually provide the service; the clinician evaluates the results and modifies the procedures.

Contact Ulcers (Contact Granuloma). Benign lesions on the posterior third of the glottal margin; possibly due to trauma, reflux, or vocally abusive behaviors; voice symptoms include low pitch, effortful phonation, and vocal fatigue.

- Do not recommend complete vocal rest or surgical treatment
- Do not recommend forced whispering
- Ask the patient to talk less
- Reduce Vocally Abusive Behaviors
- Teach the client to speak with less effort and force
- Teach relaxed phonation and speaking
- Teach the client to speak more softly
- Eliminate glottal attacks

Contingency. An interdependent relation between events or factors; in behavioral analysis and treatment, a dependent relation between antecedents, responses, the clinician's feedback to the client; includes Environmental Contingency and Genetic/Neurophysiological Contingency

Contingent Queries. Questions the clinician asks immediately following an unclear statement from the client in language therapy; lead to more specific or elaborate responses from the client.

- Ask a question immediately following an unclear response from the child (e.g., the child says "kick ball;" you ask, "who is kicking the ball?")

Continuous Airflow. A stuttering treatment target; maintaining uninterrupted airflow throughout an utterance; for procedures see Stuttering, Treatment; Treatment of Stuttering: Specific Techniques or Programs.

Continuous Reinforcement. A schedule in which every occurrence of a responses is reinforced.

- Use this schedule only in initial stage of treatment
- Gradually shift from continuous to Intermittent Reinforcement

Contrast Effect. Increase in the frequency of an undesirable response that has been kept under check by an aversive stimulus when the aversive stimulus is absent.

Contrastive Stress Drills. A treatment method used to promote both articulatory proficiency and natural prosody, especially the stress and rhythm aspects of spoken language; used in treating Apraxia of Speech (AOS) in Adults; different phrases and sentences are used to teach placing stress on different words; stressed words or terms may be used to promote articulatory proficiency or simply to vary prosodic features of speech.

In Teaching Articulatory Proficiency

- Construct phrases and sentences preferably with a single target sound in them (e.g., "My name is Peter" for /p/; "Sam did it" for /s/)
- Ask a series of questions such that the client will respond with the target phrase placing extra stress on the target word (e.g., "Is your name Tom?;" client will respond 'No, my name is *Peter*;" the client is likely to stress the word *Peter*, especially the initial sound, and thus improve the articulatory precision of /p/; similarly, ask "Tom did it?;" the client will respond "*Sam* did it")
- Reinforce the client for articulatory proficiency

In Teaching Prosodic Features

- Create a series of phrases and sentences (e.g., "Tom does not read mystery novels")
- Ask questions that will force stress on different words in target phrases and sentences (e.g., "Does Tom read *romance* novels?" may evoke "No, Tom reads *mystery* novels" "Does Tom *never* read mystery novels?" may evoke "Tom *reads* them all the time"
- Reinforce the client for varying stress on different words

Control Group. The group that does not receive treatment and hence shows no change in the target disorder or disease; part of the Group Design Strategy that helps evaluate treatment effects and efficacy.

- Select subjects randomly (Random Selection)
- Assign subjects into control and experimental groups randomly
- Alternatively, match subjects in the experimental and control groups (See Matching)
- Assess the two groups
- Withhold treatment to the control group while the experimental group receives treatment.
- Demonstrate that the control group did not change (improve) while the experimental group did

Controlled Evidence. Data that show that a particular treatment, not some other factor, was responsible for the positive changes in client's behavior; evidence gathered through controlled experimentation with either group or single-subject design strategy; one of several Treatment Selection Criteria.

Controlled Sentences. Specific sentences that contain target language features the clinician asks the child to produce; may be modeled; pictures and other clinical stimuli may be used to evoke them; less spontaneous.

Conversational Probes. Methods to assess generalized production of clinically established behaviors in conversational speech and language.

- Take a naturalistic conversational speech sample
- Direct it minimally to adequately sample the production of speech or language behaviors under probe
- Count the number of opportunities for producing the skill under probe
- Calculate the percent correct production of probed behaviors
- Give additional training at the conversational level if the adopted probe criterion is not met (e.g., 90% accuracy)
- Dismiss the client only after the criterion is met

Conversational Turn Taking. A pragmatic language skill and treatment target; often deficient in clients with language disorders; involves appropriate exchange of speaker and listener roles during conversation; for procedures, see

Language Disorders in Children; Treatment of Language Disorders: Specific Techniques or Programs.

Corrective Feedback. Response-contingent feedback from the clinician that reduces the frequency of undesirable responses of clients; frequently used in treatment.

- Give corrective feedback as soon as you detect an incorrect response
- Give Verbal Corrective Feedback ("No," "That is not correct") for all incorrect responses
- Give Nonverbal Corrective Feedback when appropriate (gestures that show disapproval of a response)
- Give Mechanical Corrective Feedback, or Biofeedback whenever possible
- Measure the frequency of incorrect responses to see if the feedback is effective
- Replace ineffective forms of corrective feedback with other, potentially more effective forms
- Minimize the use of corrective feedback by giving more positive feedback for correct responses and by Shaping complex skills

Craniocerebral Trauma. The same as Traumatic Brain Injury.

Criteria for Making Clinical Decisions. Rules to make various clinical judgments; includes such treatment related rules as when to model, when to stop modeling, and when a behavior is considered trained.

- Model most target behaviors for most clients, especially in the initial stages
- Discontinue modeling when the client gives five consecutively correct, imitated responses
- Reinstate modeling if errors persist
- Consider an exemplar of a target behavior trained when the client gives 10 consecutively correct responses
- Consider a behavior tentatively trained when the client gives 90% correct responses on untrained exemplars on an intermixed probe

- Consider a behavior trained when the client gives 90% or better correct responses in conversational speech produced in extraclinical situations

Cultural Diversity and Treatment Procedures: See Ethnocultural Variables in Treatment.

Cysts. Acquired or congenital, fluid-filled lesions of the larynx caused by trauma; can occur contralaterally to a unilateral Vocal Nodule; usually unilateral; treatment is surgery.

Deaf. A person whose hearing impairment is severe enough to prevent normal oral language acquisition, production, and comprehension with the help of audition; profound hearing loss that exceeds 90 dB HL.

Deblocking. A technique used in treating clients with aphasia; uses an intact response to one kind of stimulus to deblock a deficient or absent response to another kind of stimulus (e.g., visual stimuli to which the client responds appropriately may be used in promoting a deficient or nonexistent responses to auditory stimuli; for the procedure, see Aphasia, Treatment; Treatment of Naming: Targets and Techniques.

Dedicated Systems of Augmentative Communication. Computers designed and built exclusively for augmentative communication.

Delayed Auditory Feedback (DAF). A procedure in which a speaker's speech is fed back to his or her ears through headphones after a delay; most speakers slow their speech down under DAF; technique is used in reducing the speech rate in persons who stutter or clutter and those who have dysarthria; see Cluttering; Dysarthria; Stuttering; Treatment of Stuttering: Specific Techniques or Programs.

- Select one of the several DAF machines available on the market
- Experiment with different durations of delay that induce speech that is free from stuttering or cluttering or a speech rate that improves intelligibility in dysarthric speakers
- Train and stabilize the target speech skills with the selected delay
- Fade DAF and shape the normal rate and prosody

Deletion Processes. A group of phonological processes in which one or more consonants or a syllable in a word is deleted or omitted; in phonological treatment, the target is to eliminate such processes; major deletion processes include:

- ***Cluster reduction:*** one or more consonants are deleted in a cluster of consonants (e.g., bu for *blue*)
- ***Initial consonant deletion:*** omission of an initial consonant of a syllable (e.g., ink for *sink*)
- ***Final consonant deletion:*** omission of a final consonant (e.g., goo for *good*)
- ***Syllable deletion:*** omission of a syllable (e.g., medo for *tomato*)

Demands and Capacities Model (DCM). A theory of stuttering which states that when the environmental demands made on a child to produce and sustain fluency exceeds the child's capacity to do so, stuttering results; treatment involves reducing the demands and gradually increasing the child's fluency skills; for procedures see Stuttering, Treatment; Treatment of Stuttering: Specific Techniques or Programs: Stuttering Prevention: A Clinical Method.

Dementia. An acquired neurological Syndrome associated in most cases with persistent or progressive deterioration in intellectual and communicative functions and general behavior; sustained over a period of months or years; examples include dementia due to Alzheimer's Disease, Huntington's Disease, Parkinson's Disease, or vascular disease; dementia is static in a few cases and reversible in 10 to 20% of the cases; in most cases, treatment is concerned with behavioral and clinical management because the disease is progressive and the effects irreversible; both the client and his or her family need treatment.

General Clinical Management of Dementia

- Establish a simple routine
- Design reminders or prompters to manage the memory problems:
  - teach the client to use portable alarms that remind appointments, scheduled activities
  - give written instructions on daily living chores (closing the windows, locking the doors, turning the stoves off); teach the client to follow the instructions

  - train staff members in healthcare facilities to give frequent and systematic reminders to the clients
  - teach the client to use self-monitoring devices
  - post signs about activities and routines and train the client to use them
- Teach clients to make a written list of *what to do* every day
- Teach the client to keep personal belongings (keys, clothing items, eye glasses, pens) in a specific, invariable place
- Teach the client to keep related objects together (e.g., paper and pencil; socks and shoes; coffee and sugar)
- Train the client to carry a card that contains the name, address, telephone of a family member and a healthcare professional
- Teach the client to wear a bracelet that contains personal identification
- Instruct the client to exploit his or her strengths to compensate for weaknesses (e.g., writing down everything when memory tends to fail)
- Teach clients to ignore relatively minor problems (word-finding difficulties)

Management Strategies for Patient's Caregivers, Including Family Members. Ask all those who care for and regularly interact with the client to:

- Approach the client slowly
- Establish eye contact before speaking
- Supplement speech with gestures, smile, posture
- Speak clearly and directly
- Speak in simple terms
- Specify referents for speech
- Record problems that occur
- Ask yes/no questions
- Ask either/or questions
- Ask short questions
- Ask simple questions
- Repeat questions if necessary
- Avoid asking open-ended questions

- Not to use too many pronouns
- Be redundant, repeat, and restate
- Talk about familiar and concrete topics and directly observable objects
- Use photographs and drawings to improve understanding
- Avoid the use of analogies
- Restate and paraphrase when the client has not comprehended
- Use touch
- Say good-bye or other departing signals
- Observe what conditions aggravate the client's behavioral problems and try to avoid or reduce those conditions
- Look for physical reasons for emotional outbursts (e.g. pain, side effects of medication)
- Look for early warning signs of emotional or aggressive outbursts (e.g., body rigidity, a certain look, crying)
- Eliminate stimuli and situations that trigger emotional and aggressive responses; engage the client in a distracting activity
- Reduce difficult demands
- Limit choices about food and clothing so that the client has fewer choices to make and reduced chances to get confused

Bayles, K. A., & Kaszniak, A. W. (1987). *Communication and cognition in normal aging and dementia*. Austin, TX: PRO-ED.

Brookshire, R. H. (1992). *An introduction to neurogenic communication disorders* (4th ed.). St. Louis, MO: Mosby Year Book.

Lubinski, R. (1991). *Dementia and communication*. Philadelphia: B. C. Decker.

Demonstration. A stimulus procedure used in treatment; usually preceded by instructions on how to produce a target response.

- Model a response for the client
- Show how the response is produced (e.g., how /k/ is produced)
- Give maximum feedback (use a mirror if necessary)
- Reinforce the correct response or an approximation of it

Denasality (Hyponasality). Lack of nasal resonance on nasal sounds; a disorder of resonance; treatment procedures under Voice Disorders; Treatment of Disorders of Resonance.

Dependent Variables. Effects studied by scientists; target behaviors taught to clients and pupils; contrasted with Independent Variables.

Deteriorating Baselines. Baselines of a progressively worsening problem; desirable behaviors (e.g., fluency) that are lower each time they are measured; require immediate treatment; an exception to the rule that in a treatment evaluation study, intervention should be started only after baselines are stable.

- Measure baselines repeatedly
- If the desirable behavior shows a consistent worsening (or the undesirable behavior shows a consistent increase) across baseline sessions, initiate treatment immediately

Determinism. A philosophical position that nothing happens without a cause; basis of modern science, whose goal is to explain events by finding their causes.

Developmental Apraxia of Speech (DAS). A speech disorder in children that shares some common characteristics with Apraxia of Speech (AOS) in Adults, but without documented neuropathology; primarily an articulatory (phonologic) disorder characterized by sensorimotor problems in positioning and sequentially moving muscles for the volitional production of speech; associated with prosodic problems; not caused by muscle weakness or neuromuscular slowness; presumed to be a disorder of motor programming for speech; controversial because of the absence of neuropathology; little or no controlled treatment efficacy data; most treatment programs are only suggestive.

Motor-Programming Approaches

- Plan on providing intensive treatment to children with DAS
- Use multiple repetitions of speech movements

- Use extensive drill; stress sequence of movements involved in speech production
- Determine the need for auditory discrimination training
- Progress hierarchically from easy to difficult tasks
  - determine at what level the child will respond (phonemes, syllables, words)
  - concentrate on vowels and consonants that children produce early
  - teach consonants that are visible
  - teach phonemes that occur often
  - teach voiceless consonants before voiced consonants
- Provide multimodality input on sound productions (visual, auditory, kinesthetic, tactile)
- Teach Self-Control (Self-Monitoring) Skills
- Reduce the speech rate if necessary
- Manipulate prosodic features within the treatment program; use such programs as Contrastive Stress Drills; if necessary increase pause durations between words
- Use techniques of treating Articulation And Phonological Disorders

Hall, P. K., Jordan, L. S., & Robin, D. A. (1993). *Developmental apraxia of speech: Theory and clinical practice*. Austin, TX: Pro-Ed.

Diagnosis. A clinical activity designed to find causes of diseases or disorders, especially in medicine; in communicative disorders, diagnosis often is aimed at describing and assessing the degree of severity of disorders; requires precise and reliable measurement of communicative behaviors; often means the same as Assessment.

- Take a case history
- Interview the client
- Screen hearing
- Conduct an orofacial examination
- Administer standardized tests that are culturally and linguistically appropriate for the client
- Design and use client-specific procedures
- Take a comprehensive speech-language sample

- Analyze the results and make a clinical judgment
- Write a diagnostic report which includes recommendations

Differential Reinforcement. (a) The method of establishing discriminated responding by reinforcing a response in the presence of one stimulus and not reinforcing the same response in the presence of another stimulus; (b) an indirect method of response reduction by increasing another, desirable behavior; specific techniques include Differential Reinforcement of Alternative Behaviors (DRA), Differential Reinforcement of Incompatible Behaviors (DRI), Differential Reinforcement of Low Rates of Behaviors (DRL), and Differential Reinforcement of Other Behaviors (DRO).

Differential Reinforcement of Alternative Behaviors (DRA). One of the Indirect Methods of Response Reduction in which an undesirable behavior is reduced by reinforcing a specified desirable behavior that serves the same function as the one to be reduced; also known as Functional Equivalence Training.

- Find out what function (purpose) the undesirable behavior to be reduced seems to serve (e.g., fussing in treatment sessions may mean that the child finds the task too difficult and cannot request help)
- Select a behavior that is a desirable alternative to the behavior to be reduced (e.g., the response "help me," if the child could make it, may serve the same function as fussing)
- Reinforce the production of the alternative, desirable response (e.g., teach the child to say "help me" instead of fussing)

Differential Reinforcement of Incompatible Behaviors (DRI). One of the Indirect Methods of Response Reduction in which an undesirable behavior is reduced by reinforcing a behavior that is incompatible with the behavior targeted for reduction.

- Specify the behavior to be reduced (e.g., leaving the chair and walking in the therapy room)

- Specify a behavior that is incompatible (e.g., sitting quietly and looking at the stimulus items presented)
- Systematically reinforce the child (for sitting quietly and looking at the stimulus items)
- Suspend training on the target communicative skill for a while if necessary and until the sitting behavior is stabilized

Differential Reinforcement of Low Rates of Responding (DRL). One of the Indirect Methods of Response Reduction in which an undesirable behavior is reduced by reinforcing its progressively lower frequency of occurrence; the method shapes down an undesirable behavior.

- Specify the undesirable behavior to be reduced (e.g., interrupting treatment by irrelevant questions)
- Specify an acceptable level of the undesirable behavior (e.g., two questions in a 10-min.-period)
- Reinforce the client for not exceeding the set level ("Good! You asked only two questions during the last 10 minutes!")
- Specify a new, more stringent criterion in successive stages until the behavior is eliminated or kept to a minimum

Differential Reinforcement of Other Behaviors (DRO). One of the Indirect Methods of Response Reduction in which an undesirable behavior is reduced by reinforcing any one of many unspecified behaviors; the behavior that will not receive reinforcement is clearly stated.

- Specify the undesirable behavior to be reduced (e.g., leaving the chair and walking around)
- Tell the client that he or she will not receive reinforcers for that behavior; also tell that he or she will receive a reinforcer as long as the undesirable behavior is not exhibited
- Periodically reinforce the child for not exhibiting the undesirable behavior (perhaps for sitting quietly, reading, coloring, working on other assignments, but none specified as the response to be reinforced)

Digital Manipulation. Physical manipulation of the larynx during voice therapy; for the procedure, see Voice disorders: Specific Normal Voice Facilitating Techniques.

Diplophonia. Double voice resulting from differential vibration of the two folds or vibration of both the true and false vocal folds.

Direct Language Treatment Approaches. Clinician-planned and implemented language treatment with specified target behaviors; structured treatment sessions; requires that the child first imitate and then spontaneously produce the selected target behaviors; described under Language Disorders in Children; Treatment of Language Disorders: Specific Techniques or Programs.

Direct Methods of Response Reduction. Procedures to reduce undesirable behaviors by directly placing a contingency on them; contrasted with Indirect Methods of Response Reduction.

- Specify the undesirable behavior to be reduced
- Place one of the following contingencies on it:
  - Corrective Feedback (e.g., say "No")
  - Time-Out (say "stop," turn your face away for 5 sec and then reestablish eye contact and resume conversation)
  - Response Cost (take a token back contingent on every incorrect response)
  - Extinction (ignore the response)
  - Imposition of Work (ask a child who disrupts your stimulus materials to organize them for you)

Discrete Trials. Structured treatment or probe trials that are temporally separated and provide discretely measured opportunities for producing responses; useful in establishing target skills but not efficient in promoting generalized and maintained production; include Baseline Evoked Trials, Baseline Modeled Trials, Treatment Evoked Trials, and Treatment Modeled Trials.

Discrimination. A behavioral process of establishing different responses to different stimuli; opposite of generalization; needed to teach such discriminated responding as plural words to plural stimuli and singular words to singular stimuli.

Distinctive Features. Unique characteristics of phonemes that distinguish one phoneme from the other; the system is binary in that a feature is scored as 1 if it is a characteristic of a phoneme and as 0 if it is not; may be used in economically describing errors of articulation and their changes in treatment (see treatment of Articulation and Phonological Disorders: Treatment of Articulation and Phonological Disorders: Specific Techniques or Programs); Chomsky-Halle's major distinctive features include the following:

- Vocalic (voiced sounds)
- Consonant (sounds characterized by vocal tract constriction)
- High (sounds produced with elevated tongue position)
- Back (sounds produced with the tongue retracted)
- Low (sounds produced with lowered tongue position)
- Anterior (sounds produced with point of constriction being relatively anterior)
- Coronal (sounds produced with raised tongue blade)
- Rounded (sounds produced with lips rounded)
- Tensed (sounds produced with relatively greater muscle tension)
- Voiced (sounds produced with vocal fold vibration)
- Continuant (sounds that can be produced in a continuous manner)
- Nasal (sounds produced with nasal resonance)
- Strident (sounds produced by forcing airstream through a small opening)

Dysarthria. A group of motor speech disorders resulting from disturbed muscular control of the speech mechanism due to damage of the peripheral or central nervous system; oral communication problems due to weakness, incoordination, or paralysis of speech musculature; classified into types including Ataxic Dysarthria, Flaccid Dysarthria, Hyperkinetic Dysarthria, Hypokinetic Dysarthria, Mixed Dysarthria, Spastic Dysarthria, and Unilateral Upper Motor Neuron Dysarthria.

General Guidelines on Treatment

- Set the treatment goal as increased efficiency, effectiveness, and naturalness of communication

- Be fully knowledgeable about the medical, surgical, pharmacological, and prosthetic management, their limitations, and how they affect communication training
- Consider the complicating medical condition, associated conditions, and their prognosis in planning treatment
- Finalize the treatment plan only after a thorough discussion with family members
- Consider the client's environment and typical communication partners in planning treatment goals and procedures
- Exploit the client's strengths (e.g., residual physiological support)
- Start management early
- Provide treatment frequently
- Organize sessions to move from easy to difficult tasks
- End sessions with success
- Spend time on activities that focus on improvement of communication
- Increase physiologic support for speech initially
- Use intensive, systematic, and extensive drill
- Use modeling (followed by imitation), shaping, prompting, fading, differential reinforcement, and other proven behavioral management procedures
- Use phonetic placement and its variations
- Provide instruction and demonstration
- Teach self correction, self-evaluation, and self-monitoring skills
- Provide immediate, specific, and social and natural feedback
- Use instrumental feedback or biofeedback when necessary
- Use consistent and variable practice
- Emphasize accuracy initially
- As accuracy is achieved, emphasize rate increase
- Restore lost function to the extent possible
- Teach compensatory behaviors for lost or reduced functions
- Reduce dependence on lost or reduced function
- Increase muscle strength
- Consider not recommending treatment if the motor speech disorder creates no disability or handicap
- Implement alternative or augmentative communication systems, if necessary

Provide counseling and support

- Teach the client to inform listener at the outset of an interaction how to effectively communicate with him or her (e.g., demonstrating use of an Alphabet Board)
- Train the client to set the context and topic before beginning a conversation
- Train the client to modify content and length of utterances
- Teach the client to monitor listener comprehension
- Teach significant others to modify physical environment, be active listeners, and maximize their own hearing and visual acuity
- Teach the client and significant others to maintain eye contact, establish effective communication strategies, and determine methods of feedback

General Treatment Goals for Clients with Dysarthria

- Modification of respiration
- Modification of phonation
- Modification of resonance
- Modification of articulation
- Modification of prosody

General Treatment Procedures

Because of the variability of dysarthria, its subclassifications, and varied neuropathology, select a particular treatment target and strategy only when a careful assessment of the client's clinical problems justifies it; some techniques produce temporary effects; others are contraindicated for certain clients; many are suggested based on clinical experience and lack controlled experimental evidence to support their routine use; continue to use a technique only when it produces a clear and positive effect on the client's behavior.

Modification of Respiration

- Train consistent production of subglottal air pressure; use manometer or air pressure transducer
- Train maximum vowel prolongation
- Shape production of longer phrases and sentences

- Teach controlled exhalation
- Teach the client to push, pull, or bear down during speech or nonspeech tasks
- Use manual push on abdomen
- Find a normal or an unusual posture that promotes respiratory support and teach it (e.g., some clients' speech improves in supine position)
- Let the client use neck and trunk braces if helpful
- Use adjustable beds and wheelchairs to make postural adjustments
- Use girdles and wraps around the abdominal area to increase muscle strength for respiration
- Use an Expiratory Board to stabilize the abdominal muscles for respiration
- Teach the client to inhale more deeply and exhale slowly and with greater force during speech
- Train the client to terminate speech earlier during exhalation

- Discuss with medical staff the need, effects, and effectiveness of medical treatments including Laryngoplasty, Teflon or Collagen Injection, Recurrent Laryngeal Nerve Resection, Botulinum Toxin Injection, and pharmacological measures; consider them in the total management of the client and in treating communication disorders
- Use biofeedback devices to give the client immediate feedback on vocal intensity to effect changes in excessive or too little loudness
- Train the client with too soft voice in using a portable amplification system
- Train aphonic clients in the use of Artificial Larynx
- Ask clients with aberrant neck movements or neck muscle weakness to wear Neck Braces
- Teach Effortful Closure Techniques for clients with vocal cord paralysis (e.g., pulling or pushing while phonating)
- Teach the client to initiate phonation at beginning of exhalation

- Teach the client to turn head toward weak side during speech; try digital manipulation of the thyroid cartilage to increase loudness; be aware of temporary effects of these
- Try relaxation exercises and laryngeal massage to increase loudness
- Teach the client to tilt head back, initiate speech after a deep inhalation, and increase pitch to reduce strained voice quality
- Teach the client with vocal cord hyperadduction to initiate phonation with breathy onset or a sigh

Modification of Resonance

- Discuss with medical staff the need, effects, and effectiveness of medical treatments including pharyngeal flap surgery, Teflon injection into the posterior pharyngeal wall, and palatal lift prosthesis to treat velopharyngeal incompetence
- Provide feedback on nasal airflow and hypernasality by using a mirror, nasal flow transducer, or a Nasendoscope
- Train the client to open the mouth wider to increase oral resonance and vocal intensity
- Use nasal obturator or nose clip; have the client speak in the supine position; be aware of temporary improvement

Modification of Articulation

- Discuss with medical staff the need, effects, and effectiveness of medical treatments including Neural Anastomosis, botulinum toxin (Botox) injection to orofacial or mandibular muscles to decrease abnormal movements, and pharmacological treatment in relation to communication training.
- Analyze the error patterns and their potential reasons before developing a treatment program
- Encourage the client to assume the best posture for good articulation
- Use a bite block to improve jaw control and strength

- Use the behavioral methods to treat articulation disorders with clients for whom articulatory modification is a main target
  - provide instructions and demonstrations
  - simplify the task, use shaping
  - model frequently
  - use phonetic placement techniques
  - reduce speech rate to improve intelligibility
  - ask the client to exaggerate the production of medial and final consonants
  - give immediate feedback
  - use minimal contrast pairs (e.g., *peet-beet; stop-top*)
  - teach self-monitoring skills
  - modify techniques in light of data
  - move from simpler level of training to more complex levels
- Experiment with such stretching exercises as sustained jaw opening and maximum tongue protrusion to see if they help improve articulation
- Use electromyographic biofeedback to reduce hypertonicity and spasm of speech muscles
- Teach compensatory articulatory movements (e.g., use of tongue blade to make sounds normally made with tongue tip)
- Use meaningful stimuli when possible
- Use intelligibility drills
  - ask the client to read texts or describe pictures you are not familiar with
  - retell what you hear
  - let the client work on improving his or her articulation to promote better understanding on your part

To improve speech rate

- Use such prosthetic devices as Delayed Auditory Feedback (DAF), a Pacing Board, an Alphabet Board, or a metronome
- Use hand or finger tapping

- Provide visual feedback from computer or storage oscilloscope
- Use rhythmic or metered cueing; point to words in a passage in rhythmic or metered fashion
- Modify pauses in speech

Modification of Prosody

- Reduce the speech rate
  - use Delayed Auditory Feedback
  - use computer programs that generate cursor movements to pace the rate of speech
  - experiment with hand or finger tapping; be aware that some clients accelerate their tapping and the speech rate
  - use a Pacing Board to reduce the rate
  - use Alphabet Board Supplementation (ask the client to point to the first letter of each word to be spoken on an alphabet board)
  - use instructions, modeling, shaping, and differential reinforcement to slow the rate
- Modify pitch with the help of instruction, modeling, differential feedback, or with the help of such instruments as VisiPitch®; be aware that direct work on pitch modification may not be needed in many cases because of successful modification of rate, intonation, and stress
- Shape louder speech through behavioral methods of modeling, shaping, and differential reinforcement of greater inhalation, increased laryngeal adduction, and wider mouth opening
- Teach the client to chunk utterances into natural syntactic units to promote more natural sounding speech
- Increase breath control to extend breath groups
- Use Contrastive Stress Tasks (sentences with the same words that change meaning when different words are stressed)
- Teach client to signal stress by using other means (e.g., prolongation of syllables or pausing before a stressed word)
- Teach the client to vary the number of words per breath group

- Begin treatment with structured tasks and make transition to conversational speech
- Teach client to self-monitor

Duffy, J. R. (1995). *Motor speech disorders.* St. Louis, MO: C. V. Mosby.

Johns, D. F. (Ed.). (1985). *Clinical management of neurogenic communicative disorders*. Boston: Little, Brown

Yorkston, K. M., Beukelman, D. R., & Bell, K. R. (1988). *Clinical management of dysarthric speakers*. Austin, TX: Pro-Ed.

Dysfluencies. Behaviors that interrupt fluency; measured in diagnosing Stuttering; specific forms include repetitions of sounds, syllables, words and phrases; prolongations of sounds and articulatory postures; inter- and intralexical pauses; interjections of syllables, words, and phrases; revisions; and incomplete phrases.

Dysphagia. Disorders of swallowing; associated with many medical conditions including neuromuscular disorders and cancer and its surgical treatment of structures involved in swallowing; may occur at any age although more common in the elderly; includes:

- ***Disorders of mastication.*** Problems in chewing food; may be due to reduced range of movement by the tongue and the mandible, reduced buccal tension, and poor alignment of mandible and maxilla.
- ***Disorders of the preparatory phase of the swallow.*** Problems in collecting the masticated food to form a bolus as a preparation for swallow; may be due to problems in labial closure, tongue movement and coordination, appropriate holding of the bolus in the mouth (e.g., holding it in the front of the mouth), and reduced oral sensitivity.
- ***Disorders of the oral phase of the swallow.*** Problems in the tongue movement to initiate the voluntary aspect of the swallow and in passing the food over the base of the tongue; by the end of the phase, the bolus will have reached the faucial arch area; problems due to tongue thrust, reduced tongue tension and movement, and reduced buccal tension.

- ***Disorders of the pharyngeal stage of the swallow.*** Problems in propelling the bolus through the pharynx and into the P-E segment; may be due to delayed or absent swallowing reflex, inadequate velopharyngeal closure, reduced pharyngeal Peristalsis, pharyngeal paralysis, laryngeal movement disorders, and so forth.
- ***Disorders of the esophageal phase of the swallow.*** Problems in passing the bolus through the cricopharyngeus muscle and past the 7th cervical vertebra; due to many muscular and other problems including weak cricopharyngeus, esophageal Peristalsis, and esophageal obstruction (e.g., by a tumor).

Treatment of Dysphagia. Management of swallowing problems by direct, indirect, and medical procedures.

General Guidelines

- Discuss the swallowing process and the treatment procedure to be implemented
- Give written instructions to the patient and describe the steps to be followed
- Ask the patient to first practice swallow (without solid or liquid food)
- Introduce only a small amount of food during direct treatment
- Show the client the amount to be swallowed
- Instruct the patient to cough to clear the airway and reinforce the client's coughs
- Initiate indirect treatment if the patient aspirates 10% of each bolus and the direct methods do not progressively reduce aspirations (intake of food into lungs); be aware that only radiographic data show aspiration
- Concentrate on increasing muscle control during indirect treatment
- Reduce distraction during treatment

Direct Treatment of Dysphagia. Treating swallowing disorders by placing food or liquid in the patient's mouth and then shaping and reinforcing swallowing behaviors.

Disorders of mastication

- Instruct the patient with limited lateral tongue movement to mash food by pressing tongue against the hard palate or by keeping the food on the more mobile side of the tongue
- Teach the patient with reduced buccal tension to:
  - apply a gentle pressure with the one hand on the damaged cheek to increase cheek tension
  - put food on the normal or stronger side
  - keep the head tilted to the stronger side to maintain food on that side
- Teach the patient with limited lateral movement of the mandible to mash food by pressing the tongue against the palate
- Design a Palate Reshaping Prosthesis for the patient with limited vertical tongue movement when indirect treatment (exercises) fail
- Gradually reshape the prosthesis by reducing its size as the patient's vertical tongue movements improve

Disorders of the preparatory phase of the swallow.

- Teach the patient with problems in forming and holding the bolus due to reduced tongue movement and coordination to
  - tilt the head forward to keep the food in front the mouth until ready to swallow
  - tilt the head back to promote the swallow
  - consciously hold the bolus in the anterior or middle portion of the mouth

- Teach the patient with reduced oral sensitivity to
  - place food on the side of the oral cavity with better sensitivity
  - better appreciate the placement of food by placing cold or spicy food in the mouth

Disorders of the oral phase of the swallow

- Teach the patient who has developed a tongue thrust to:
  - place the tongue on the alveolar ridge and initiate a swallow with an upward and backward motion
  - compensate by placing food at the back of the tongue and then to initiate a swallow
- Teach the patient with reduced tongue elevation to:
  - compensate by placing food posteriorly in the oral cavity
  - place the straw almost at the level of the faucial arches to help swallow liquid
  - tilt the head back and let gravity push the food from the oral cavity into the pharynx
  - use the Supraglottic Swallow Maneuver to voluntarily protect the airway, if aspiration is a concern
- Teach the patient with disorganized anterior to posterior tongue movement to
  - hold the Bolus against the palate with the tongue
  - begin the swallow with a strong, single posterior motion of the tongue
- Teach the patient with a scarred tongue to
  - place food behind the scarring
  - tilt the head posteriorly to allow gravity to help with oral transit

Disorders of the pharyngeal stage of the swallow

- Teach the patient with delayed or absent swallowing reflex to compensate by:
  - tilting the head forward while swallowing
  - limiting the amount of Bolus that does not overflow into the open airway

- counsel the family about the delay in initiating the swallow reflex; ask them to allow that much extra time for each swallow
- Teach the patient with reduced peristalsis such compensatory behaviors as:
  - switching between liquid and semisolid swallows so that the liquid swallows help clear the pharynx
  - taking only liquids or semisolids
  - initiating dry swallows after each swallow of food to clear the pharynx
  - the Supraglottic Swallow Maneuver
- Teach the patient with unilateral pharyngeal paralysis such compensatory behaviors as
  - turning the head toward the affected side to close the pyriform sinus on the affected side and to direct the food down the normal side
  - tilting the head toward the stronger side if the patient has a unilateral paralysis in lingual function and the pharynx
  - the Supraglottic Swallow Maneuver
  - washing away residual thicker food with liquid swallows
- Ask the patients with cervical osteophyte to limit their diet to semisolid or liquid food until surgery corrects the problem and the patient recovers
- Teach the patient with a scarred pharyngeal wall the same compensatory behaviors used for the patient with unilateral pharyngeal paralysis
- Teach the patient with reduced laryngeal elevation to clear the throat after each swallow
  - use the Supraglottic Swallow Maneuver if residual material needs to be removed from the pharynx
- Teach the patient with reduced laryngeal closure to
  - use the Supraglottic Swallow Maneuver
  - tilt the head forward while swallowing
  - turn the head to the side that is not functioning properly

- place pressure on the thyroid cartilage on the damaged side to improve closure

Disorders of the esophageal phase of the swallow

Do not attempt to treat as these are handled medically

Logemann, J. (1983). *Evaluation and treatment of swallowing disorders*. San Diego, CA: College-Hill Press.

Indirect Treatment for Dysphagia. Treatment of swallowing problems using exercises designed to improve the muscle functioning; does not involve food.

Oral-motor control exercises

- Treat the patient with reduced range of tongue movements with such exercises as the following; ask the patient to:
  - open the mouth as wide as possible and raise the tongue in front as high as possible; hold the tongue for a second, and then lower it
  - raise the posterior part of the tongue as far as possible; hold it for 1 second, and then lower it
  - continue with the stretching exercises for 5–10 times in a session, for 3–4 minutes
  - repeat the set of exercises 5–10 times per day
- Increase the patient's buccal tension by asking the patient to
  - stretch the lips as tightly as possible and say "e"
  - round the lips tightly and say "o"
  - rapidly alternate between "e" and "o"
- Instruct the patient with limited lateral movement of the mandible to
  - keep the jaw open as widely as possible and hold this position for about 1 second
  - open and move the jaw sideways and hold the extended position for 1 second
  - make circular jaw movements
  - provide Manual Guidance to move the jaw in the desired directions

    - stop the task if any pain is experienced
- Treat the patient with limited tongue resistance by asking the patient to
    - push the tongue against a tongue depressor and hold the pressure for 1 second
    - push the tongue against the tongue blade, in an upward, forward, and sideways direction; hold the pressure for 1 second
- Shape more firm lip closure by asking the patient with problems in lip closure to:
    - stretch the lips for 1 second to stimulate the production of /i/; increase the duration gradually
    - pucker the lips tightly for 1 second initially; increase duration gradually
    - close the lips tightly for one second; increase the duration gradually; provide Manual Guidance if necessary
    - close the lips around a spoon or an object; reduce the size of the object as the patient's lip closure improves
    - to hold the lips together for 1 minute once a lip seal is achieved; increase the duration gradually
    - repeat the exercises 10 times per day
    - ask the patient to close the lips around a tongue depressor
    - maintain lip closure when you or the patient tries to open them
- Treat the patient with bolus control problems by asking the person to grossly manipulate materials by
    - holding a flexible licorice whip in the mouth, with one end on the patient's tongue and the other end in the clinician's hand
    - keeping the licorice stick between the palate and the tongue
    - moving the licorice stick from side to side with the tongue

- moving the licorice stick forward and backward with the tongue, and then report where the licorice stick is
- reporting when gross movement of the licorice stick is achieved
- moving the licorice stick in a circular motion starting from the center of the mouth
- chewing a piece of gum as manipulation capabilities improve

- Treat the patient with bolus control problems who has learned to grossly manipulate materials by
  - placing a small bolus of paste consistency on the tongue
  - asking the patient to move the bolus around in the mouth
  - telling the patient not to spread the bolus around in the mouth
  - asking the patient not to lose the bolus
  - instructing the patient to cup the tongue around the bolus
  - expectorating the bolus once the task is complete (inspect the mouth for residue)
  - varying the consistency of the bolus, once success is achieved
  - introducing one-third of a teaspoon of liquid to the patient's mouth once success is achieved with the paste
- Treat the patient with bolus propulsion problems through posterior bolus propulsion exercises
  - place a long wad of gauze that is dipped in fruit juice in the patient's mouth
  - hold one end of the gauze
  - ask the patient to use the tongue to push the gauze up and back

Stimulating the swallow reflex

- Hold a small, long-handled laryngeal mirror in ice water for about 10 seconds

- Place the laryngeal mirror at the base of the anterior faucial arch
- Repeat this light contact 5–10 times
- Observe the likely rise of the thyroid cartilage, the twitching of the soft palate, and a slight movement of the faucial arches
- Ask the patient to swallow after the stimulation without food
- After repeating light contact stimulation some 5–10 times, release a small amount of liquid into the patient's mouth with a pipette and ask the patient to swallow by saying "Now."
- Repeat stimulation exercises four to five times daily for weeks to a month in the case of patients with severely impaired swallow reflex
- Shape swallowing once the reflex begins to trigger by progressively larger amounts of food and food with greater consistency

Improving adduction of tissues at the top of the airway

- Teach lifting and pushing exercises to improve laryngeal adduction to protect the airway during swallowing; ask the patient to
  - sit on a chair and hold his or her breath as tightly as possible
  - use both hands and push down, or pull up on the chair, while holding the breath for 5 seconds
  - use only one hand while pushing down or pulling up on the chair and to try and produce clear voice with each trial; repeat this exercise 5 times
  - use Hard Glottal Attack and repeat "ah" five times
  - repeat the exercises three times in succession, 5–10 times a day for 1 week
  - lift or push with simultaneous voicing; use both hands, pull on a chair, and use prolonged phonation

- use Hard Glottal Attack, commence phonation on "ah," and sustain phonation with smooth voice quality for 5–10 seconds
- practice a Pseudo Supraglottic Swallow; instruct the patient to inhale, hold the breath, and use a strong cough

Medical Treatment of Dysphagia. Use of such surgical procedures as the following to treat dysphagia:

Cricopharyngeal Myotomy. gical procedure of splitting the cricopharyngeal muscle from top to bottom to keep a permanently open sphincter for swallowing; fibers of the inferior constrictor above and the esophageal musculature below also may be slit; eating may be resumed within about a week; recommended for patients with Parkinson's disease, amyotrophic lateral sclerosis, and oculopharyngeal dystrophy whose main problem is cricopharyngeal dysfunction.

Esophagostomy. A nonoral, surgical feeding method for dysphagic patients who cannot tolerate oral feeding; insertion of a feeding tube into the esophagus and stomach through a hole (stoma) surgically created through cervical esophagus.

Gastrostomy. A nonoral, surgical feeding method for dysphagic patients who cannot tolerate oral feeding; insertion of a feeding tube into the stomach through an opening in the abdomen; blended table food is directly transported to the stomach.

Nasogastric Feeding. A nonoral feeding method for dysphagic patients who cannot tolerate oral feeding; a tube inserted through the nose, pharynx, and esophagus into the stomach feeds the patient.

Pharyngostomy. A nonoral, surgical feeding method for dysphagic patients who cannot tolerate oral feeding; insertion of a feeding tube into the esophagus and stomach through a hole (stoma) surgically created through the pharynx.

Teflon Injection into Vocal Folds. A surgical implant method to improve airway closure during swallowing in dysphagic patients by adding implanted muscle mass that will help close the airway; Teflon may be injected to a normal or reconstructed vocal cord or any remaining tissue on top of the airway.

Logemann, J. (1983). *Evaluation and treatment of swallowing disorders.* San Diego, CA: College-Hill Press,.

Dysphonia. A general term that means disordered voice; any voice disorder with the exception of Aphonia.

Dystonia. Movements that are repetitive, slow, twisting, writhing, and flexing. Uncontrolled adductor and abductor laryngeal spasms occur; voice is breathy, strained, and hoarse.

Echolalia. Parrot-like repetition of what others speak; a major characteristic of autism.

Ear Training. The same as Auditory Discrimination Training or Perceptual Training.

Effectiveness of Treatment. Assurance that treatment, not some other factor, was responsible for the positive changes documented in a client under treatment; requires controlled evidence gathered through clinical experimentation.

Effortful Closure Techniques. Behavioral treatment techniques to promote laryngeal abduction for clients with unilateral or bilateral vocal cord paralysis or weakness; the client is taught to grunt, cough, push, lift, and pull to achieve closure of the folds and then phonate.

Electronic Communication Systems. Methods of augmentative communication for persons with limited or no oral speech; also known as electronic gestural-assisted communication strategies, these systems use electronic devices with a switching mechanism to activate a message, control electronic system, and a display that shows the message; used in teaching Augmentative Communication, Gestural-Assisted (Aided).

Electronic Device for Alaryngeal Speech (Electrolarynx). Hand-held electronic instruments that generate sound which is used by persons who have undergone Laryngectomy to produce alaryngeal speech; for rehabilitation procedures, see Laryngectomy; Treatment Procedures: Laryngectomy.

Electronic Gestural-assisted Communication Strategies. The same as Electronic Communication Systems.

Elicited Aggression. Aggressive behavior directed against any object or person when an aversive stimulus (as in operant punishment procedures) is delivered; not necessarily directed against the person delivering the aversive stimulus; a potential undesirable side-effect of punishment.

Empirical Validity. Credibility or truthfulness of statements based on research data; assurance that treatment procedures have been shown to be effective through experimentation involving clients (as against logical arguments or scholarly speculation); a criterion for treatment selection.

Empiricism. A philosophical position that statements must be supported by observational or experimental evidence; basis of modern science; contrasted with Nativism or Rationalism.

Environmental Contingency. Interdependent relation between antecedents, response, and the consequences the responses generate and thus help maintain those responses; environmental events that shape and sustain behaviors; the treatment variable in behavioral approach; contrasted with Genetic/Neurophysiological Contingency with which it interacts.

Escape. A behavior that reduces or terminates an aversive event and hence increases in frequency; typically leads to avoidance; often maladaptive as in a stutterer's avoidance of speaking situations; reduction of avoidance may be a clinical goal.

- Work on eliminating the aversiveness of the event by teaching the needed, alternative skill (e.g., increased fluency in speaking situation)
- In gradual steps, encourage the client to come in contact with the aversive event (avoided speaking situation)
- Reinforce the approach behavior

Escape Extinction. A procedure to reduce negatively reinforced behaviors by blocking an escape and thus preventing negative reinforcement for it; a response reduction strategy.

- Prevent the occurrence of an undesirable response (e.g., crawling under the table) exhibited to escape from aversiveness (e.g., training trials)
- Physically restrain the child every time an attempt is made to leave the chair to prevent reinforcement of escape behavior

- Measure the frequency of attempts to crawl; if there is no reduction, use a different technique

Ethnocultural Variables in Treatment. Variables related to individual's cultural, ethnic, and other personal variables that may affect treatment of communicative disorders.

- Select assessment procedures that are ethnoculturally relevant
- Select treatment stimulus materials that are ethnoculturally appropriate
- Select treatment procedures that are known to have ethnocultural generality
- Gather systematic client performance data on treatment procedures that are of unknown ethnocultural generality
- Modify treatment procedures in light of the performance data and the client's ethnocultural background

Event Structures. Sequentially organized, familiar events taken from daily life and routinized to teach language structures to children; for procedures, see Language Disorders in Children; Treatment of Language Disorders: Specific Techniques or Programs.

Evoked Trials. Structured opportunities to produce a response when the clinician does not model; part of the discrete trial procedure; often used in the beginning stages of treatment; include Baseline Evoked Trials and Treatment Evoked Trials.

Exemplar. A response that illustrates a target behavior; it may be words, phrases, sentences, gestures, and so forth; an individual stimulus item designed to evoke specific target response; generally, teaching a few exemplars is sufficient to generate other exemplars of the same behavior.

Expansions. A language treatment technique in which a client's incomplete or telegraphic utterances are expanded into grammatically more complete productions; for procedures, see Language Disorders in Children; Treatment of Language Disorders: Specific Techniques or Programs.

Experiment. A controlled condition in which an independent variable (such as treatment) is manipulated to produce changes in a dependent variable (production of speech or language); a means of establishing cause-effect relations; needed to establish treatment effects; may use the Group Design Strategy or the Single-Subject Design Strategy.

Experimental Group. In a clinical experiment, the group that receives treatment and hence shows changes in skills taught; part of the Group Design Strategy for establishing treatment effectiveness; contrasted with a Control Group.

- Select subjects randomly (Random Selection)
- Assign subjects into control and experimental groups randomly
- Alternatively, match subjects in the experimental and control groups (Matching)
- Assess the experimental and control groups to make sure they are equal
- Treat the experimental group while withholding treatment to the control group
- Demonstrate that the experimental group changed (improved) while the control group did not

Expiratory Board. A prosthetic devise used to improve respiratory muscle strength for speech; client pulls a board attached to wheelchair toward his or her abdomen and leans against it to stabilize the muscles.

Explanation. A statement that describes an event and points out its causes; based on experimental evidence on cause-effect relations; a goal of science.

Exclusion Time-Out. Response-contingent exclusion of a person from a reinforcing environment; a variety of Direct Methods of Response Reduction; a form of Time-Out.

- Contingent on an undesirable behavior, remove the child from the stream of activities (e.g., make the child sit outside the classroom or in a corner)
- Bring the child back to the stream of activities after a brief period of time

Extension. A language treatment method in which the clinician makes comments on the child's utterances to add additional meaning; for procedures, see Language Disorders in Children; Treatment of Language Disorders: Specific Techniques or Programs.

Extinction (of Automatically Reinforced Behaviors). The procedure of terminating automatic reinforcers for responses to be reduced; one of the Direct Methods of Response Reduction; especially useful in reducing self-stimulatory behaviors of clients who are autistic, profoundly mentally retarded, or brain injured.

- Determine the sensory consequence of the undesirable behavior to be reduced (noise from banging on the table; stimulation from banging the head)
- Reduce or eliminate the sensory stimulation derived from the behavior to be reduced (cover the table with soft material or make the child wear padded helmet)

Extinction (of Negatively Reinforced Behaviors). The procedure of terminating negative reinforcers for responses to be reduced; one of the Direct Methods of Response Reduction; also known as Escape Extinction; appropriate to reduce such behaviors as crawling under the table or leaving the chair and walking around because treatment trials are aversive and the behavior provides escape and negative reinforcement.

- Physically prevent the behavior
- Continue to present treatment trials

Extinction (of Positively Reinforced Behaviors). The procedure of terminating positive reinforcers for responses to be reduced; one of the Direct Methods of Response

Reduction; appropriate to reduce such behaviors as crying maintained by reinforcement; should ***not*** be used to reduce aggressive, self-destructive, and generally disruptive behaviors or those that are due to physical pain and discomfort.

- At the very outset of the behavior to be reduced, tell the client that you will pay attention only when that behavior stops
- Pay no more attention until the behavior stops; turn your back and sit motionless; do not try to use other means of stopping the behavior
- Do not be unnerved when the behavior initially intensifies (Extinction Burst)
- Pay immediate attention when the behavior subsides or stops

Extinction Burst. A sudden, initial, and temporary increase in responses at the beginning of extinction; not a reason to abandon extinction when it is appropriately chosen.

Extraclinical Settings (Training In). Training given in such nonclinical settings as play ground, classroom, home, and other places; essential part of Maintenance Strategy; training is less formal, involving spontaneous, functional communication; often administered by such significant others as teachers, family members, and friends.

Eye Contact. Looking at the listener's face during conversation; a pragmatic language intervention target; for procedures, see Language Disorders in Children; Treatment of Language Disorders, Specific Techniques or Programs.

Facilitated Communication. A technique of language treatment for children with autism and others with severe language impairment in which a facilitator maintains physical contact with the hand, wrist, or elbow of the client to facilitate writing, typing, or pointing on a message board; controlled studies have produced negative evidence; results suggest that the facilitator may be the source of the messages typed; the American-Speech-Language-Hearing Association is not convinced of its effectiveness and recommends additional research; the American Psychological Association and the Association for Behavior Analysis have concluded that the method is ineffective and invalid.

Factorial Stimulus Generalization. Generalized production of unreinforced responses given in relation to new stimuli, settings, and audience; the most complex form of stimulus generalization.

- Use a variety of stimuli to evoke target behaviors
- Vary treatment settings
- Arrange different conversational partners for the client
- Probe for factorial stimulus generalization

Fading. A method of reducing the controlling power of such special stimuli as modeling while still maintaining the target responses the stimuli evoke.

- Reduce the frequency of the special stimulus (e.g., modeling) gradually
- Reduce the intensity of the stimulus (e.g., present Prompts in progressively softer voice)
- Present only a partial stimulus (as in Partial Modeling)
- Make the stimulus progressively more subtle (e.g., make the hand gesture given to slow down the speech of a person who stutters less conspicuous)
- Make a mechanical stimulus nonfunctional (e.g., turn off a microphone that the client still holds, or turn off a computer screen that remains in front of the client)

- Increase the distance from the client and the special stimulus in graded steps (move the microphone or the computer screen away from the client)

First Words. The first few words a child typically acquires; language treatment targets for young children who are nearly nonverbal.

- Select child-specific words
- Select the names of family members, child's favorite toys (car, doll), food items (milk, juice, candy), clothing items (sock, shoe), action verbs (come, go, walk), simple adjectives (big, small), animals (kitty, doggie), household objects (pen, book, spoon, chair, table), and words from similar categories
- Use the structured, Direct Language Treatment Approaches if the child is nearly nonverbal and has attention deficit:
  - use the Discrete Trials
- Use indirect language stimulation if the child interacts well and can concentrate on loosely structured treatment activities; use a play-oriented situation:
  - frequently model the target word productions
  - use the Mand-Model approach
  - use the Incidental Teaching Method
- Train parents to stimulate language at home; teach parents to:
  - have the child label an item before handing it
  - read stories to the child and have the child name pictures
  - ask questions about the pictures (e.g., "how does the kitty go?")
- Give training in varied contexts and probe for generalized productions
- Move on to teaching Phrases (Word Combinations)

Fixed Interval Schedule (FI). An intermittent schedule of reinforcement in which an invariable time duration separates opportunities to earn reinforcers; the first response made after the interval is reinforced; responses made during the interval are not reinforced; limited use in treating communicative disorders.

Fixed Ratio Schedule (FR). A schedule of reinforcement in which a certain number of responses are required to earn a reinforcer; an FR1 in which every response is reinforced is a continuous schedule; schedules greater than 1 are intermittent; frequently used in treatment sessions.

- Specify the schedule to the client ("I will give you a token every time you say it correctly")
- Reinforce according to the specified schedule

Flaccid Dysarthria. A type of motor speech disorder; its neuropathology is damage to the motor units of cranial or spinal nerves that supply speech muscles (lower motor neuron involvement); speech problems caused mostly by muscle weakness and Hypotonia; constellation of speech disorders dependent on the specific nerve that is affected, but include breathy voice quality, hypernasality, and imprecise production of consonants; select appropriate treatment targets and procedures described under Dysarthria; in addition, consider the following that apply especially to flaccid dysarthria:

- Target increased muscle strength or compensation for weakness as the main treatment outcome
- Modify respiratory behaviors
  - use pushing/pulling exercises to increase respiratory support
  - use postural adjustments
  - teach the client to use deep inhalation and controlled exhalation
- Increase loudness
- Increase breath group durations
- Increase the number of words per breath group
- Consider Teflon®/collagen injections for vocal fold adduction
- Improve resonance and velopharyngeal functioning
- Consider palatal lift prostheses and pharyngeal flap surgery

- Use a bite block to improve tongue and lip movement for speech

Duffy, J. R. (1995). *Motor speech disorders.* St. Louis, MO: C. V. Mosby.

Johns, D. F. (Ed.). (1985). *Clinical management of neurogenic communicative disorders.* Boston: Little, Brown

Yorkston, K. M., Beukelman, D. R., & Bell, K. R. (1988). *Clinical management of dysarthric speakers.* Austin, TX: PRO-ED.

Fluency. An aspect of speech and language production; quality or state of being fluent.

Fluency Reinforcement Techniques. Reducing stuttering by increasing fluency; fluent intervals or fluent utterances may be reinforced; for procedures see Stuttering, Treatment; Treatment of Stuttering: Specific Techniques or Programs.

Fluency Shaping Techniques. A collection of stuttering treatment techniques based on the assumption that normal-sounding fluency should be the intervention goal; contrasted with Fluent Stuttering: Van Riper's Approach described under Stuttering, Treatment; Treatment of Stuttering: Specific Techniques or Programs.

Fluent Speech. Speech that is smooth, flowing, effortless, and rapid within acceptable limits; negatively defined, it is speech that does not contain excessive amounts of pauses, repetitions, sound and silent prolongations, interjections, and other forms of dysfluencies; speech that is not produced with excessive effort and struggle.

Fluent Stuttering: Van Riper's Approach. A stuttering treatment approach based on the assumption that reduced abnormality of stuttering, not fluent speech, is a realistic goal for most persons who stutter; for procedures see Stuttering, Treatment; Treatment of Stuttering: Specific Techniques or Programs.

Fluency Disorders. Speech disorders characterized by excessive amounts of dysfluencies or excessive duration of dysfluencies or both, and speech that is produced with excessive amounts of struggle and effort (Stuttering); speech that is characterized by excessively fast rate, indistinct articulation, and possibly language formulation problems (Cluttering); impaired fluency due to Neurogenic Fluency Disorders; Stuttering is the most researched, and more frequently diagnosed and treated fluency disorder in the United States.

Follow-Up. Assessment of response maintenance subsequent to dismissal from treatment; done according to a schedule (such as 3 months after dismissal or at 6-month intervals).

- Set up a schedule with decreasing frequency (e.g., twice in the first six months of dismissal, the next follow-up after a year, the next after two years)
- Take a speech-language sample
- Measure the frequency of the target behaviors (production of clinically established speech sounds, language structures, fluency or dysfluency, vocal qualities, etc.)
- Calculate the percent correct use of the clinically established target behaviors
- Give Booster Treatment if the target behaviors are below the previously set criterion (such as 90% accuracy)

Functional Equivalence Training. An indirect method of reducing an undesirable behavior by reinforcing a desirable behavior that serves the same function as the undesirable behavior; the same as the Differential Reinforcement of Alternative Behaviors (DRA).

Generality (of treatment). The applicability of a treatment procedure in a wide range of situations involving other clients and clinicians; demonstrated through Replication of treatment efficacy research; a Treatment Selection Criterion.

Generalization. A declining rate of unreinforced responses in the presence of untrained stimuli; a temporary, intermediate goal of treatment; includes Verbal Stimulus Generalization, Physical Setting Generalization, Audience Generalization, Factorial Stimulus Generalization, and Response Generalization; each may be promoted with specific techniques.

Generalized Production. Production of clinically established behaviors in relation to new stimuli, new audiences, and in new situations; measured through Probes.

Genetic/Neurophysiological Contingency. The interdependent relation between genetic and neurophysiological variables that determine or influence behaviors; contingency that interacts with Environmental Contingency.

Gentle Phonatory Onset. A stuttering treatment target; initiating voice in a gentle, soft, easy, relaxed manner; also a treatment target in treating hard glottal attack; for procedures see Stuttering, Treatment; Treatment of Stuttering: Specific Techniques or Programs; and Voice Disorders, Treatment of Voice Disorders.

Gestural Communication. Method of communication that supplements oral communication with smiles and a variety of other facial expressions, body movements including shoulder shrugging, hand movements, pantomime, pointing, and head nodding or shaking; part of normal oral communication; in gestural communication, they play a more crucial role of communicating the speaker's messages; gestural communication may be unaided as in smiling or hand movements; or aided, as in gestures combined with a communication board; procedures described under Augmentative

Communication, Gestural (unaided) and Augmentative Communication, Gestural-Assisted (aided).

Glottal Fry. A normal voice register that may occur at the end of sentences; very low-pitched vocalization that may sound like the popping of popcorn; also called vocal fry.

Gradient of Generalization. Progressively decreasing, unreinforced response rate as a stimulus is varied on a given dimension, resulting in a curve that approximates the bell-shaped curve; the reason why generalization is not a final treatment goal.

Gradual Increase in Length and Complexity of Utterances (GILCU). A component of the Monterey Fluency Program; for procedures see Stuttering, Treatment; Treatment of Stuttering: Specific Techniques or Programs.

Granulovacuolar Degeneration. A build-up of fluid-filled vacuoles and granular remains within nerve cells; a basic neuropathology of Alzheimer's Disease and found in some normal elderly people.

Group Design Strategy. A research strategy in which the experimental treatment effect or efficacy is demonstrated by treating individuals in one group (the experimental group) and not treating individuals in another, comparable group (control group); one of two strategies for treatment evaluation; contrasted with Single-Subject Design Strategy.

- Select a sample of subjects randomly from a defined population
- Randomly assign subjects to an experimental and a control group
- If random selection and assignment are not possible, match subjects in the two groups on relevant variables
- Treat subjects in the experimental group
- Withhold treatment from the control group
- If the experimental group improves while the control group did not, conclude that the treatment was effective

Hard of Hearing. Persons who have reduced hearing acuity but nonetheless are able to acquire, produce, and comprehend language primarily with the help of audition; may use amplification and visual cues to understand speech.

Hard Glottal Attack. Abrupt voice initiation with too much stress on individual words; words of a sentence sound too separated; a vocally abusive behavior.

- Teach gentle, relaxed, easy onset of phonation
- Teach the client to blend words initially
- Use the Chewing technique, Whisper-Phonation, the Chant-Talk, and the Yawn-Sigh, all described under Voice Disorders, Specific Normal Voice Facilitating Techniques.
- Contrast the easy-onset production with a hard-onset production

Harshness. Voice quality that results from excessive laryngeal tension, effort, and constriction.

- Use relaxation to reduce vocal tension
- Teach soft, easy contact of the vocal folds
- Teach gentle onset of phonation
- Use a combination of Specific Normal Voice Facilitating Techniques described under Voice Disorders

Hearing Impairment. Reduced hearing acuity; a hearing level that is greater than 25 dB HL in case of adults and 15 dB HL in case of young children in the process of language acquisition; includes the Hard of Hearing and the Deaf; classified as shown under Hearing Loss; oral speech and language disorders are a common concomitant of hearing impairment, especially deafness; mostly, the treatment procedures for Language Disorders in Children, Articulation and Phonological Disorders, and Voice Disorders are applicable with the following special considerations:

General Guidelines

- Begin speech and language stimulation training as early as possible

- Have the child under appropriate medical and audiological management
- Get the family involved from the very beginning in speech and language stimulation activities
- Have the child fitted with an individual hearing aid
- Work closely with the educators and special educators, especially the educator of the deaf
- Train family members to work with the child at home conducting sessions that parallel yours

Teaching Oral Language

- Begin oral language training as early as possible
- Teach the basic words initially; select functional words
- Teach phrases and sentence structures subsequently
- Pay special attention to teaching grammatic morphemes as they are especially difficult for children with hearing impairment
- Pay special attention to pragmatic use of language as it is especially difficult for children with hearing impairment; teach such skills as Topic Initiation, Topic Maintenance, and Turn Taking described under Language Disorders in Children; Treatment of Language Disorders: Specific Techniques or Programs.
- Pay special attention to teaching abstract terms, terms with dual meanings, and the meaning of proverbs as they are especially difficult for children with hearing impairment
- Pay special attention to teaching synonyms and antonyms as they are especially difficult for children with hearing impairment
- Use visual cues in all training sessions
- Refer to specialists who can teach such nonverbal communication systems as American Sign Language if the clients, families, or both prefer

Teaching Articulatory Skills

Give ample visual cues in teaching speech sound production

- Use such procedures as the Phonetic Placement Method
- Pay special attention to fricatives, stops, and affricates as these are especially difficult for children with hearing impairment
- Teach voiced and voiceless sound distinctions
- Use mechanical visual feedback

Treating Voice Disorders

- Use the standard techniques described under Voice Disorders
- Use mechanical, visual feedback with such instruments as VisiPitch®
- Modify such abnormal voice qualities as harshness, hoarseness, stridency, and monotone
- Modify resonance disorders; modify both hypernasality and hyponasality

Treating Prosodic Problems

- Teach smooth flow of speech
- Reduce pauses that may be too frequent and placed inappropriately
- Teach normal intonation
- Teach appropriate breath control to improve phrasing
- Modify the pitch
- Modify loudness

Hearing Loss. Roughly the same as Hearing Impairment; classified as follows:

- Mild hearing loss: 15–40 dB HL
- Moderate hearing loss: 41–70 dB HL
- Severe hearing loss: 71–90 dB HL
- Profound hearing loss: 90 dB and higher

High Probability Behaviors. Behaviors of high frequency that can reinforce those of low frequency; an effective treatment method to increase low frequency treatment targets.

- Identify behaviors your client exhibits frequently (e.g., listening to music, watching television, or skiing)

- Design a method by which you in the treatment sessions and the family members at home can control opportunities for those behaviors
- Give tokens in treatment sessions for producing the low-frequency communicative skills
- Let the client accumulate the tokens and exchange them for opportunities to engage in the high-probability behaviors (brief periods of listening to music in treatment sessions, watching television at home, or going on ski trips)

Hoarseness. Voice quality that results from leakage of air and aperiodic vibration of the vocal folds; pitch may be too low; any condition that changes the mass and size of the vocal folds, including vocal nodules, may cause hoarseness of voice.

- Obtain a medical evaluation and clearance before starting voice therapy
- Modify the vocally abusive behaviors
- Use a combination of Specific Normal Voice Facilitating Techniques, described under Voice Disorders.

Huntington's Disease. An Autosomal Dominant, degenerative neurological disease; caused by neuronal loss in the caudate nucleus and putamen along with diffuse neuronal loss in the cortex; symptoms include Choreiform Movements and Dementia; associated with motor speech disorders and language impairment; general management procedures described under Dementia.

Hyperadduction. Closure of vocal folds with excessive force and tension.

- Teach laryngeal relaxation
- Teach breathy onset of phonation
- Teach gentle, relaxed, easy phonatory onset
- Massage the larynx
- Use such other specific normal voice facilitation techniques as the Yawn-Sigh technique and the Chewing Technique described under Voice Disorders; Specific Normal Voice Facilitating Techniques.

Hyperkinetic Dysarthria. A type of motor speech disorder; its neuropathology is damage to basal ganglia (extrapyramidal system) resulting in rapid involuntary movements and variable muscle tone; may affect all aspects of speech, but a dominant symptom is prosodic disturbances; specific problems include prolonged intervals, variable rate, monopitch, loudness variations, inappropriate silences, imprecise consonants, and distorted vowels; most effective treatment is medical; select appropriate treatment targets and procedures described under Dysarthria, Treatment; in addition, consider the following that apply especially to hyperkinetic dysarthria:

- Use a Bite Block to inhibit or reduce interfering jaw movement in clients with mandibular Dystonia
- Use postural adjustments to facilitate speech production
- Slow down the rate of speech
- Teach slower rate and increased vocal pitch when appropriate

Duffy, J. R. (1995). *Motor speech disorders.* St. Louis, MO: C. V. Mosby.

Johns, D. F. (Ed.). (1985). *Clinical management of neurogenic communicative disorders.* Boston: Little, Brown

Yorkston, K. M., Beukelman, D. R., & Bell, K. R. (1988). *Clinical management of dysarthric speakers.* Austin, TX: PRO-ED.

Hypernasality. Nasal resonance on non-nasal speech sounds; a resonance disorder; intervention described under Voice Disorders; Treatment of Disorders of Resonance.

Hypertonia. Excessive tone or tension.

Hypoadduction. Inadequate approximation of vocal folds; results in breathiness and weak voice; often associated with neurological involvement.

- Elicit coughing, grunting, throat clearing, and laughing to improve Adduction
- Use Digital Manipulation of the Larynx described under Voice Disorders; Specific Normal Voice Facilitating Tech-

niques; use this technique along with pressure applied to the abdominal muscles to increase subglottic pressure

- Teach pushing, pulling, and lifting exercises and combine them with phonation

Hyponasality. Reduced or absent nasal resonance in the production of nasal sounds; the same as Denasality; intervention described under Voice Disorders; Treatment of Disorders of Resonance.

Hypotonia. Reduced tone or tension.

Hypokinetic Dysarthria. A type of motor speech disorder; its neuropathology is damage to basal ganglia (extrapyramidal system) resulting in slow movement, limited range of movement, and rigidity; may affect all aspects of speech, but especially voice, articulation, and prosody; specific problems include monopitch, monoloudness, reduced stress, imprecise consonants, inappropriate silences, harsh and breathy voice, and short rushes of speech. select appropriate treatment targets and procedures described under Dysarthria, Treatment; in addition, consider the following that apply especially to hypokinetic dysarthria:

- Use rate-control for clients who speak rapidly
  - use delayed auditory feedback and pacing boards if necessary
  - shape a slower rate of speech
- Use voice therapy techniques to increase vocal loudness and to decrease breathiness
- Use voice amplifiers to increase loudness
- Decrease breathiness

Duffy, J. R. (1995). *Motor speech disorders.* St. Louis, MO: C. V. Mosby.

Johns, D. F. (Ed.). (1985). *Clinical management of neurogenic communicative disorders.* Boston: Little, Brown

Yorkston, K. M., Beukelman, D. R., & Bell, K. R. (1988). *Clinical management of dysarthric speakers.* Austin, TX: Pro-Ed.

Iconic Symbols. A symbol that looks like the object it is supposed to represent; used in teaching Augmentative Communication, Gestural-Assisted (aided); easier to learn than Noniconic Symbols.

Ideographic Symbols. Graphic representation of ideas; more abstract than pictographic symbols; may be line drawings; used in teaching Augmentative Communication, Gestural-Assisted (aided).

IEPs (Individualized Education Programs). Child-specific intervention programs designed for children with disabilities or special needs served in public grade schools.

- Assess the child's strengths and weaknesses
- Write an IEP for each child you serve
- State the short- and long-term intervention objectives in measurable terms
- Describe the frequency and duration of your intervention sessions
- Specify the amount of time the child will spend in regular classroom
- Specify the intervention initiation and termination dates
- Justify the need for your services (use the school district's guidelines in determining service eligibility)
- Specify the names of special education or other professionals who also will serve the child
- Hold an IEP meeting to finalize the intervention plan and to get the signatures of all attending, including those of the parents

IFSPs (Individualized Family Service Plans). Special education programs designed for children with disabilities in the age range of birth through 2 years and their family members.

- Develop a plan similar to IEPs
- Include information on the family's needs and strengths
- Orient the plan toward family involvement

Imitation. A response that follows a modeled stimulus and takes the same or similar form of its stimulus; frequently used in the beginning stages of treatment of most if not all communicative disorders; Modeling is the treatment technique to evoke imitation.

Imitation of Aversive Control. Use of aversive methods to control others by persons who were subjected to aversive control themselves; a potential, undesirable side-effect of punishment procedures.

Imposition of Work. One of the Direct Methods of Response Reduction in which an undesirable behavior is reduced by immediately imposing work designed to reduce or eliminate the negative effects of that behavior; also known as overcorrection; has two components: Restitution and positive practice.

Restitution

- Immediately following an undesirable behavior (e.g., throwing toys around), ask the child to neutralize the effects of that behavior (pick up the toys)
- Ask the child to go beyond neutralizing the effects of his or her behavior by improving the situation (ask the child to clean-up the mess created by another child or put the toys on a shelf)

Positive Practice

- Ask the child to practice an incompatible, appropriate behavior repeatedly without reinforcement (ask the child to organize your stimulus materials)

Improvement. Documented positive changes in the client's behaviors compared to initial assessment or baseline performance; not the same as Effectiveness of Treatment which requires controlled evidence.

Incidental Teaching Method. A naturalistic language treatment method that uses everyday verbal interactions to teach functional communication skills; procedure described under Language Disorders in Children; Treatment of Language Disorders: Specific Techniques or Programs.

Incompatible Behaviors. Behaviors that cannot be produced simultaneously, such as sitting and walking; used to reduce certain undesirable behaviors; targets in the Differential Reinforcement of Incompatible Behaviors (DRI).

Independent Variables. Hypothesized or demonstrated causes of events scientists investigate; treatment methods clinicians use; anything a clinician does that affects the client's behavior; contrasted with Dependent Variables.

Indirect Language Stimulation. A collection of somewhat varied, naturalistic, unstructured or minimally structured language stimulation procedures based on play activities; for procedures, see Language Disorders in Children; Treatment of Language Disorders: Specific Techniques or Programs.

Indirect Methods of Response Reduction. Reducing certain behaviors by increasing other behaviors; indirect because no contingency is placed on behaviors to be decreased; include Differential Reinforcement of Alternative Behavior, Differential Reinforcement of Incompatible Behavior, Differential Reinforcement of Low Rates of Responding, and Differential Reinforcement of Other Behavior.

Informative Feedback. Information provided to the client on his or her performance levels that reinforces clinical target skills; may be verbal or mechanical; contrasted with Mechanical Corrective Feedback, Nonverbal Corrective Feedback, or Verbal Corrective Feedback in which the information provided is specific to the wrong responses to be decreased.

Verbal

- Periodically, tell the client how well he or she is doing ("You have improved to 85% today")
- Show and describe charts and graphs that depict increases in target skills

Mechanical

- Display positive changes and improvement data on computer monitors and other display devices

Inhalation Method. A method of air intake to produce esophageal speech; for procedures, see Laryngectomy; *Treat Esophageal Speech*.

Inhalation Phonation. A technique of voice therapy to evoke true vocal fold vibration in clients who are aphonic; for procedures, see Voice Disorders, Specific Normal Voice Facilitating Techniques.

Injection Method. A method of air intake to produce esophageal speech; for procedures, see Laryngectomy; *Treat Esophageal Speech*.

Initial Response. The first, simplified component of a target response used in Shaping.

Instructions. Verbal stimuli that promote the production of target responses; often used in treatment sessions; combined with Demonstrations, Modeling, and Manual Guidance (as in Phonetic Placement Method)

- Design instructions that clarify the target behavior for the client
- Simplify your instructions and tailor them to the individual client
- Write your instructions and practice their delivery, but deliver them naturally; do not read them
- Repeat instructions until the client understands them
- Combine them with demonstrations, modeling, and manual guidance

Intention Tremor. Tremor that is absent during periods of rest, but manifests itself during voluntary movements

Interfering Behaviors. Behaviors that interrupt the treatment process; includes such behaviors as leaving the chair, asking irrelevant questions during treatment, crying, wiggling in the chair, and inattentiveness; sometimes a priority focus for clinical intervention because speech-language behaviors cannot be trained unless such interfering behaviors are reduced or eliminated.

- Use one of the Differential Reinforcement procedures to increase the alternative desirable behaviors which will then reduce the interfering behaviors

Intermediate Response. Responses other than the initial and the final responses used in Shaping a target skill.

Intermittent Reinforcement. Several schedules of reinforcement in which only some responses or responses produced with specified delay are reinforced; produces stronger response rates than Continuous Reinforcement; includes the Fixed Ratio, Fixed Interval, Variable Ratio, and Variable Interval Schedules; useful in promoting response maintenance over time; to be used in the intermediate and final strategies of treatment.

Intermixed Probes. Procedures used to assess generalized production of a trained skill by alternating trained and untrained stimulus items.

- Prepare a Probe Recording Sheet on which you have alternated trained and untrained exemplars; have at least 10 untrained exemplars
- Present a trained exemplar on the first trial; reinforce the correct production
- Present an untrained exemplar on the second trial; provide no reinforcement or corrective feedback
- Alternate trained and untrained exemplars on the subsequent trials
- Calculate the percent correct probe responses based only on responses given to the untrained exemplars
- Give additional training when an adopted probe criterion is not met (e.g., 90% accuracy)
- Move on to next level of training or to new target behaviors when the criterion is met

Intraverbal Generalization. Stimulus and response generalization within forms of verbal behaviors; primarily includes expansions of language skills acquired under treatment.

Intubation Granuloma. A lesion of the larynx that occurs at or near the vocal process of the arytenoid because of trauma caused by the insertion, positioning, or removal of an endotracheal tube; treatment is surgical; no voice therapy except for vocal rest.

Isolated Therapy Model. A special education service delivery model in which children are taken out of the classroom for special instruction, including speech-language instruction; the same as the Pull-out Therapy Model.

Isolation Time-out. Response-contingent removal of a person from a reinforcing environment and placing him or her in a nonreinforcing environment; a variation of Time-Out.

Joint Action Routines or Interactions. A child language intervention method in which repetitive, routinized activities are used; similar to Script Therapy or may be a variation of it; for procedures, see Language Disorders in Children; Treatment of Language Disorders: Specific Techniques or Programs.

Key Word. A word in which a generally misarticulated sound is correctly produced; needed to implement the Paired-Stimuli Approach described under Articulation and Phonological Disorders; Treatment of Articulation and Phonological Disorders: Specific Techniques or Programs.

Language-Based Classroom Model. A model of service delivery in which the speech-language pathologist is in charge of a class organized especially for students with communication disorders although some normally speaking children also may be involved; the clinician teaches these children all day or part of the day.

Language Delay in Children. Generally the same as Language Disorders in Children; except for the connotation that children with language delay are slow in learning and that they will catch up with their normally progressing peers; language disorders in children tend to persist; hence, disorders and delay are not synonyms; treatment procedures the same as those for Language Disorders in Children.

Language Disabilities in Children. Generally the same as language disorders; includes an acceptable connotation that children with language problems lack certain skills necessary to meet social and academic demands; may be used interchangeably with language disorders; treatment procedures the same as those for Language Disorders in Children.

Language Disorders in Adults. Difficulty in comprehending, formulating, and producing language; often there is a history of normally acquired and used language functions; loss of language functions often are due to physical diseases, especially neurological diseases; includes Aphasia, Apraxia, Dementia, Dysarthria, and language disorders associated with Right-Hemisphere Injury and Traumatic Brain Injury.

Language Disorders in Children. Difficulty in learning to comprehend and/or produce language in a varied group of children some of whom have associated clinical conditions while others show no such conditions; also referred to as Language Delay, Language Disabilities, Language Deviance, Language Impairment, Language-Learning Disorders, and Language Problems; the term Childhood or Congenital Aphasia is dated and controversial; the term Specific Language Impairment refers to a special group of children with language problems with no other difficulties, also controversial.

A Generic Treatment Procedure for Language Disorders in Children:

- Make a complete assessment based on an extended conversational speech and other culturally sensitive assessment tools
- Determine what the child can and cannot do with language (comprehension and production; structures the child understands and uses and those that the child does not understand or use)
- Select language intervention targets that:
  - are child-specific and ethnoculturally appropriate
  - are useful in natural settings
  - can make an immediate and socially significant difference in the child's communicative skills
  - help meet the academic and social demands the child faces
  - help expand communication skills into conversational speech in natural settings
  - are within the child's reach as judged by current performance (words, phrases, sentences, conversational speech)
- Design a Sequence of Treatment that generally moves from:
  - words to phrases
  - phrases to controlled (less spontaneous) sentences
  - controlled sentences to spontaneous conversational speech
  - treatment in clinical settings to treatment in more naturalistic settings
  - more structured sessions to progressively less structured sessions
  - continuous reinforcement to intermittent reinforcement
  - primary reinforcers to social reinforcers
  - social reinforcers to natural consequences inherent in communication
- Prepare stimulus materials for treatment
  - Select ethnoculturally appropriate, client- and target-specific stimuli that are colorful, attractive, and realistic; prefer objects to pictures

- Obtain stimuli from the child's home (the child's favorite books, toys, and objects)

Prepare a Response Recording Sheet on which:
- you can write target behaviors
- record the occurrence of each behavior

Establish Baselines of target behaviors through:
- repeated conversational language samples that help reliably document the occurrence of language targets
- a set of modeled discrete trials and a set of evoked discrete trials that (a) help capture the production of specific language targets that may not be adequately sampled in conversational speech; (b) are necessary in case of children with no or minimum conversational skills

Modeled Baseline Trial	Evoked Baseline Trial
1. Place a stimulus picture or object in front of the child or demonstrate an action or enact an event	1. Place a stimulus picture or object in front of the child or demonstrate an action or enact an event
2. Ask a question to evoke the target response	2. Ask a question to evoke the target response
3. Model the response	3. Record the response
4. Record the response	

- Calculate the percent correct baseline response rate in conversational samples and on discrete modeled and evoked trials
- Write a treatment and maintenance plan
- Establish the target behaviors; if necessary and appropriate, use the structured discrete trial method to establish the target behaviors; use modeled trials initially and then switch to evoked (nonmodeled) trials:

Modeled Training Trial	Evoked Training Trial
1. Place a stimulus picture or object in front of the child or demonstrate an action or enact an event	1. Place a stimulus picture or object in front of the child or demonstrate an action or enact an event
2. Ask a question to evoke the target response	2. Ask a question to evoke the target response
3. Model the response	3. Give feedback (positive reinforcers for correct responses and corrective feedback for incorrect responses)
4. Give feedback (positive reinforcers for correct responses and corrective feedback for incorrect resonses)	4. Record the response
5. Record the response	5. Wait for a few seconds and present the next trial
6. Wait a few seconds and present the next trial	

- Discontinue modeling when the child has given 5 consecutively correct imitated responses and move on to evoked trials (no modeling)
- Reinstate modeling if errors persist
- Fade modeling through Partial Modeling
- Initially reinforce continuously; in gradual steps reduce the amount of reinforcers by switching to intermittent schedules
- Always use social reinforcers even when using tangible reinforcers
- Fade tangible reinforcers if used
- Decrease undesirable behaviors through Response Reduction Strategies

- Train each exemplar to a training criterion of 90% correct
- Train about 4 exemplars (words, phrases, or sentences) per target behavior before you probe
- Probe for generalized production of the trained language structure; initially, use the Intermixed Probes in which you alternate trained and untrained stimuli; later, use Pure Probes on which you present only untrained stimuli.

Intermixed Probe Trials	Pure Probe Trials
1. Place a stimulus, object or event used in training; ask a question to evoke the response; reinforce or give corrective feedback; record the response on a Probe Recording sheet	1. Place a stimulus, object, or event not used in training; ask a question to evoke the response; do **not** reinforce or give corrective feedback; record the response
2. Present a stimulus, object, or event not used in training; ask a question; do **not** reinforce or give corrective feedback; record the response	2. Present another stimulus picture **not** used in training and follow the same procedure as in #1.
3. Present another stimulus used in training; use the same procedure as in #1.	3. Present at least 10 untrained stimulus events.
4. Present another stimulus not used in training and use the same procedure as in #2.	4. Calculate the percent correct probe response rate.
5. Alternate trained and untrained stimuli using the same procedures as in #1 and #2; present at least 10 untrained stimulus events; recycle the trained items.	

6. Calculate the percent correct probe response rate based only on responses given to untrained stimuli.	

- When a target behavior does not meet the intermixed probe criterion of 90% correct, provide training on additional exemplars
- When a target behavior meets the intermixed probe criterion of 90% correct on at least 10 exemplars, administer the pure probe
- If the pure probe criterion of 90% is not met for a minimum of 10 exemplars, give training on additional exemplars
- When a target behavior meets a pure probe criterion of 90% correct on at least 10 untrained exemplars:
  - begin training on a more complex response level (e.g., when the child meets 90% correct probe at the word level, shift training to the phrase level)
  - select another behavior for tainting if the training time permits
- When a pure probe criterion is met for Controlled Sentences, shift training to conversational speech in which you monitor and reinforce the production of the target structures; at this stage:
  - discard discrete trials
  - loosen the training structure
  - use more spontaneous speech
  - talk about events
  - tell stories the child retells
  - use more natural language consequences including agreement (affirmation), negation, smile, handing requested objects, meaningful responses to questions, and so forth
- Integrate Pragmatic Structures into training at the spontaneous, natural, conversational speech training level:

- teach maintenance of eye contact during conversation by prompting and reinforcing the child for doing so
- teach Topic Maintenance (described later in this section under Treatment of Language Disorders: Specific Techniques or Programs) by progressively increasing the duration for which the child talks about a topic
- teach Turn Taking (described later in this section under Treatment of Language Disorders: Specific Techniques or Programs) by reinforcing the child to alternately play the role of a listener and that of a speaker
- teach Conversational Repair (described later in this section under Treatment of Language Disorders: Specific Techniques or Programs) strategies including asking questions when statements are not understood

- Implement a maintenance procedure
  - have family members, teachers, caretakers, peers, and others observe the treatment sessions
  - train the significant others, especially the family members and teachers in evoking, prompting, and consequating target behaviors
  - have family members conduct informal therapy sessions at home and bring recorded evidence to that effect
  - ask the child's teacher to provide opportunities for communication in the classroom and to praise the child for producing targeted and other language skills
  - hold informal training sessions outside the clinic room; outside the building; in other parts of the school or campus; and at other settings to the extent practical
  - use intermittent reinforcement schedule and natural, social reinforcers
  - delay reinforcement in later stages of treatment; increase the delay in gradual steps
  - always take training to the natural conversational level
  - teach Reinforcement Priming by training the child to draw attention to his or her newly acquired communicative skills

- teach Self-Control (Self-Monitoring) by training the child to recognize and measure his or her right and wrong responses
- continue treatment until the language skills stabilize in the natural environment
- Follow-Up and provide Booster Treatment

Treatment of Language Disorders: Specific Techniques or Programs

Activity-Based Language Intervention. Treating language disorders with the help of various activities designed to promote language production; a classroom-based approach in which each child has an individualized educational plan; activities are part of classroom activities and use natural antecedents and consequences.

- Plan activities that promote the production of specific language structures in children
- Plan activities around a theme if appropriate (e.g., activities related to going on a camping trip)
- Read stories, narrate events, and sing songs about the theme; include the various language targets for the children in the class
- Ask questions about the presented information
- Forget to give needed objects during activities, leading the child to request them
- Give needed items one at a time so the child requests each of them
- Put needed things out of reach so the child asks for them
- Put needed things in a clear jar that the child can see but cannot open to gain access and hence has to request help
- Hide the child's belongings to encourage requests
- Introduce novel items (e.g., wear a funny hat) and let those who talk about it wear it
- Pause during verbal or nonverbal actions so the child will request that you continue

Bricker, D., & Cripe, J. (1992). *An activity-based approach to early intervention.* Baltimore, MD: Paul H. Brookes.

Child-Centered Approaches to Language Intervention. Play-oriented, Indirect Language Stimulation in which the clinician does not target specific language structures to teach; the clinician may arrange stimuli that are more likely to evoke language structures; uses such techniques as Reversed Imitation (clinician's imitation of the child's utterance), Expansion, Extension, Parallel-Talk, Recast, and Self-Talk (all described later in this section).

Conversational Repair. Skills of handling breakdown in communication; a pragmatic language structure and a treatment target during conversational skill training; refers to such skills as asking questions when messages are not clear and responding to requests for clarification.

Teach the child to request clarifications from a speaker

Play the role of a speaker who makes ambiguous or unclear statements:

- Make ambiguous statements (e.g., say "Give me the car" when you have displayed several toy cars)
- Wait for the child to request clarification
- If the child does not request clarification and responds anyway (e.g., picks up one of the cars), say "No"
- Wait for the child to request clarification
- If the child does not request clarification, model a response for the child (e.g., "When you are not sure, I want you to ask me 'What do you mean?' OK?")
- Make another ambiguous statement
- Immediately model the request for clarification for the child
- Reinforce the child for imitating the request for clarification (e.g., "What do you mean?")
- Make another ambiguous statement
- Prompt (not model) a request for clarification (e.g., "What do you ask me?")

- Reinforce the child for asking for clarification (e.g., "What do you mean?")
- Introduce varied ambiguous statements
- Fade modeling and prompting
- Train parents in teaching the child to request for clarification
- Probe the generalized repair skill by presenting untrained messages
- Continue training until a set probe criterion (such as 90% accuracy in responding with the target skill) is met

Teach the child to vary the expressions when requested by a listener who does not understand

Play the role of a listener who does not fully understand the expressions of the child:

- Ask the child to repeat
- Ask the child "What do you mean?"
- Tell the child "I do not understand"
- Negate a child's utterance so the child will clarify by assertion ("You did not go on the roller coaster 20 times did you?"; the child might say "No, I went on it two times")
- Model the clarified statement by modifying what the child said ("You mean you want on the roller coaster two times, right?")
- Rephrase the child's utterance into a question and say it with a rising intonation ("You went on the roller coaster 20 times?")
- Model different ways of saying the same thing
- Ask the child to say it differently; reinforce varied phrases or sentences
- Periodically stop responding (e.g., to the child's request) to prompt the child to rephrase
- Train parents to prompt the child to vary expressions and to reinforce the child for compliance
- Probe the generalized repair skill by presenting untrained messages

- Continue training until a set probe criterion (such as 90% accuracy in responding with the target skill) is met

Conversational Skill. A language skill in maintaining a dialogue with one or more partners; an intervention goal for all clients with language disorders; collection of skills that include Topic Initiation, Topic Maintenance, and Turn Taking (all described later in this section).

- Use Peer Modeling (described later in this section); recruit peers who have good conversational skills to model those skills to the client
- Train the peers to model and have the client participate in conversation
- Closely monitor the behaviors of the peer models and the client
- Train peer models to be the hosts of a mock talk show
- Ask open-ended questions (you or the peer model)
- Ask follow-up questions (you or the peer model)
- Prompt the peer and the client for appropriate behaviors
- Train the client to ask questions
- Reinforce the client for new topic initiations, appropriate turn taking, and topic maintenance; if necessary, train these skills separately
- Show videotaped model interactions between adults, between children, and between children and adults
- Let the children analyze the tapes
- Let the children recreate what they saw on the tapes
- Train parents to conduct informal conversational skills training sessions at home

Delayed Stimulus Presentation. A child language intervention procedure in which the clinician delays providing such special stimuli as modeling for about 15 seconds to see if the child responds without such stimuli; provides the stimuli only when the child does not respond within the time limit.

- Establish joint attention regarding a stimulus (e.g., hold an object; establish eye contact with the child; look questioningly or expectantly)
- Do not speak for 15 seconds when the child approaches you or looks at you
- Model a mand or a name after the 15 second delay
- Give the object when the child imitates your modeling
- Give the object anyway when you have modeled 3 times and the child has not yet imitated

Direct Language Treatment Approaches. Intervention approaches in which the clinician selects specific language targets, designs a treatment environment and implements the treatment; uses specific stimuli including modeling, prompting, and manual guidance; uses explicit reinforcement contingencies; expects the child to imitate or produce specific targets upon stimulation; moves through a planned sequence of treatment stages.

Environmental Language Intervention Strategy (ELIS). A language intervention method for preschool children; developed and researched by J. D. McDonald and associates; a structured, direct treatment strategy; takes a semantic approach to teaching grammar; emphasizes generalized production at home; especially useful in training parents to conduct language stimulation sessions at home.

- Establish baselines of selected target language structures
- Structure treatment in three phases: Imitation, conversation, and play
- Introduce the three procedures in the first three individual training sessions
- Train parents to record responses and administer the treatment program at home; train them in the Management of Behavioral Contingencies

- After the first three training sessions, integrate imitation, conversation, and play into a single session
- Spend the first 15 minutes on imitative productions
  - present a nonlinguistic stimuli (throw a ball)
  - present a linguistic stimuli (e.g., "say, throw ball"
- Spend the next 15 minutes on conversational speech
  - present the same nonlinguistic stimuli
  - ask a question: (e.g., "What am I doing?")
  - model if necessary (e.g., "Say throw ball. What am I doing?"
- Spend the final 15 minutes on play activity during which the production of the target behavior is reinforced
  - let the child play with the material used in imitation and conversation
  - evoke responses from the child that are relevant to the child's actions (e.g., if the child throws the ball, ask, "What are you doing?")
- Give such positive reinforcers as tokens and verbal praise for correct responses
- Give such corrective feedback as Time-Out for incorrect productions
- Ask parents to conduct at home three weekly sessions similar to yours.
- In each session, review the records of home training and suggest modifications

MacDonald, J. D., Blott, J. P., Gordon, K., Spiegel, B., & Hartman, M. (1974). An experimental parent-assisted treatment program fro preschool language-delayed children. *Journal of Speech and Hearing Disorders, 39*, 395–415.

Event Structures in Language Treatment. Use of repetitive, sequentially organized, familiar events from daily life to teach language structures to children; an event structure may be the same as a Script used in Script Therapy (described later in this section); the two may be used in conjunction; also similar to Joint Action Routines or Interactions (described later in this section).

- Select a common event the child has repeatedly experienced (e.g., shopping for a toy, eating in a restaurant, taking part in a birthday party)
- Describe the event verbally
- Assign roles to yourself and the child (e.g., customer and the store clerk)
- Use props to act out the event
- Reverse roles and act out the events; repeat until the various language structures of interest are rehearsed
- Evoke words and phrases as you act out the event by using pauses at junctures (using the Cloze Procedure)
- Evoke increasingly complex or longer description of events
- Vary the sequence and event elements (e.g., after having worked with the event shopping for a toy, have them work with the event shopping for clothing)
- Violate expected events or sequences and let the child question you or correct you (e.g., go to the sales clerk without trying the clothes)

Expansions. Expanding a child's incomplete or telegraphic statements into grammatically more complete productions; part of Indirect Language Stimulation.

- Arrange a play situation that provides opportunities for language production
- Engage in parallel play with the child or take part in the child's activities
- Expand the child's structurally incomplete productions into more complete sentences (e.g., a boy says "baby cry" as he looks at a picture; you expand it into "the baby is crying")
- Do not ask the child to imitate your expansions

Expatiations. The same as Extensions.

Extensions. Comments on the child's utterances to add additional meaning; part of Indirect Language Stimulation; also known as Expatiations.

- Arrange a play situation that provides opportunities for language production
- Engage in parallel play with the child or take part in the child's activities
- extend the child's semantically limited productions into semantically richer, structurally complete sentences through comments, (e.g., a girl says "play ball" as she plays with a ball; you extend it to include additional meaning: "Yes, you are playing with a big ball; "You are playing with a blue ball")
- Do not ask the child to imitate your extensions

Eye Contact. A potential pragmatic communication target behavior for certain children who do not look at the listener while speaking or at the speaker while talking; potentially culturally determined; need culturally sensitive assessment and treatment.

- Target eye contact from the beginning and especially during conversational speech training
- Use simple instruction and verbal praise
- Prompt the child by saying "Look at me" before you present stimuli; when you begin to talk; when the child begins to talk
- Hold the stimulus parallel to your face so the child looks at the face and the stimulus simultaneously
- Praise the child for maintaining eye contact
- Measure the duration for which eye contact was maintained at the beginning (baseline) and throughout the treatment phase
- Fade the prompts or other cues used

Focused Stimulation. A technique of language intervention in which the clinician repeatedly models a target structure to stimulate the child to use that structure; usually a part of play activity.

- Design a play activity to focus on a particular language structure (e.g., the plural morpheme *s*)

- Collect various stimulus materials (books, cups, hats)
- Talk about the materials and repeatedly model the plural constructions ("I see two *books* here. The *books* have pictures. Here are two red *cups.* You can drink out of these *cups*. There are some *hats*. The *hats* are big")
- Do not correct the child's wrong productions
- Respond to the child's nontarget responses without insisting on the correct response (e.g., the child says "the *book* is nice;" the clinician says "Yes, the books are nice").
- Continue until the child begins to produce the target structure

Imitation of Child's Utterances. Reversed Imitation in which the clinician imitates a child's utterance during Indirect Language Stimulation; need more controlled clinical data to support its use.

Incidental Teaching Method. A Naturalistic Child Language Teaching Method (described later in this section) that uses typical, everyday verbal interactions to teach functional communication skills; the child often initiates an interactional episode; the clinician turns such episodes into opportunities to teach language; emphasis is on communication; effective when the child and the teacher interact for extended periods of time and in natural settings (e.g., in special education class rooms, institutions for the retarded and the autistic); excellent method for parents to learn and use at home.

- Select certain functional communicative skills for teaching (e.g., requests)
- Arrange therapy situations such that the child is likely to initiate a conversational exchange (e.g., place attractive toys on a shelf the child can see but cannot reach; arrange a child's clothing items or some desirable food items)
- Stay close to the arranged materials and give nonverbal cues to speak (focused attention on the child and a questioning look)

- Give a verbal cue (e.g., ask "What do you want?") only if the nonverbal prompts fail to evoke a response from the child
- Give cues that evoke more complex responses (e.g., "Ask me in a sentence" if the child gives only single word responses)
- Reinforce the child with natural consequences (e.g., "Good, here is the car;" "Very good, here is your sock;" "Fine, have some juice")
- Arrange as many such teaching episodes as possible in a day

rt, B. B., & Risley, T. R. (1982). *How to use incidental teaching for elaborating language*. Lawrence, KS: H & H Enterprises.

Indirect Language Stimulation. A collection of language stimulation procedures that are a part of play-oriented approach to teaching language disorders; also called Child-Centered Approach (described earlier in this section); less structured and more naturalistic; thought to be especially suitable for children who are passive, reluctant, or unmotivated to communicate; based on the assumption that variables observed in normally developing children are effective clinical treatment strategies; need more controlled evidence to support this approach.

- Arrange a play situation that provides opportunities for language production
- Choose the play material that are relevant for the targeted response
- Let the child lead the interaction
- Engage in parallel play with the child or take part in the child's activities
- Talk about what the child is doing, looking, playing, or talking
- Describe what you do (e.g., "See I am drawing a face; I am drawing;" Self-Talk; (described later in this section)
- Describe or comment upon what the child is doing (Parallel-Talk, described later in this section); e.g.,

you say "You are drawing, you are drawing a face, you are making a nose")

- Imitate the child's production (do *not* ask the child to imitate)
- Use Expansions (described earlier in this section); expand the child's telegraphic speech into grammatically more complete sentences (e.g., the child says "Mommy hat;" you expand this to "That is Mommy's hat")
- Use Extensions (described earlier in this section); comment on the child's utterances to add additional meaning; e.g., the child says "Mommy hat'" you say "Yes, it is a big blue hat")
- Recast (described later in this section) the child's utterances (expand the child's utterance type into a different kind of sentence; e.g., the child says "Mommy hat;" you recast it as, "Is this Mommy's hat?" or "This is not Mommy's hat")
- Do not ask the child to imitate; do not target specific language structures; do not explicitly reinforce correct productions

Integrated Functional Intervention. Approach to language treatment that emphasizes natural contexts for training, conversational speech as the main mode of training, and increased involvement of parents and significant others in promoting and maintaining language skills.

Interactive Language Development Teaching. One of Directed Language Treatment Approaches to teach syntactic structures; the clinician reads a story to the child and then asks a series of questions designed to evoke specific language structures from the child.

- Select a story that targets language concepts (e.g., camping, cooking) and specific language responses (e.g., the auxiliary is or preposition on)
- Read the story to the child
- Ask questions frequently as you tell the story to evoke specific responses; for instance, "Daddy said a bear is

coming [part of the story]. What did Daddy say?" [question to evoke the response "bear is coming"]

Lee, L., Koeningsknecht, R., & Mulhens, S. (1975). *Interactive language development teaching.* Evanston, IL: Northwestern University Press.

Joint Action Routines or Interactions. Use of repetitive, routinized activities in early language stimulation; an Indirect Language Stimulation method; similar to Script Therapy (described later in this section) or may be a variation of it.

- Use such established routines as "peek-a-boo"
- Design your own routines of action (e.g., always start treatment with telling the same short story that contains certain target language structures)
- Encourage the child to use the repetitive words, phrases, and sentences
- Reverse roles and let the child practice other language structures
- Violate a routine and let the child question you (e.g., skip the story and let the child ask "Story?" or "What about the story?")

Joint Book Reading. Systematic use of storybook reading to teach or stimulate language in children; allows for repetitive use and practice of the same phrases and concepts; helpful in establishing joint attention as well.

- Select story books that are linguistically and culturally appropriate for children under treatment
- Select books with colorful pictures
- Read the same story several times during a few sessions so that children memorize it
- Use prosodic features frequently to draw attention to specific language structures
- When the children know the story well, pause at points containing target language structures and prompt the children to supply the words, phrases, or sentences
- During different readings, pause at different junctures so the children produce different language structures

- Manipulate and vary pause locations that prompt progressively longer utterances from the children
- Ask the a child to "read" (recite from memory, but looking at the text and the pictures) and pause
- Let the other children supply the words, phrases, and sentence

Kirchner, D. (1991). Reciprocal book reading. A discourse-based intervention strategy for the child with atypical language development. In T. Gallagher (Ed.), *Pragmatics of language: Clinical practice issues* (pp 307–332). San Diego, CA: Singular Publishing Group.

Whitehurst, G., Falco, F., Lonigan, C., Fischel, J., DeBrayshe, B., Valdez-Menchaea, M., & Caulfield, M. (1988). Accelerating language development through picture-book reading. *Developmental Psychology, 24*, 552–558.

Mand-Model. A variation of the Incidental Teaching Method (described earlier in this section); uses typical adult-child interactions in a play-oriented setting to teach language.

- Select a variety of attractive toys, pictures, and other stimulus materials
- Design a naturalistic interactive situation
- Establish a joint clinician-child attention to a particular material (such as a toy); if necessary, direct the child's attention to a stimulus
- Mand a response from the child; for instance, say "Tell me what you want" or "Tell me what this is"
- Model the correct, complete response if the child fails to respond or gives a limited (e.g., single word) response
- Prompt if the child does not imitate the whole sentence you modeled (e.g., "Tell me the whole sentence")
- Praise the child for imitating or for responding correctly without modeling
- Give the material the child wants as you praise

Rogers-Warren, A., & Warren, S. (1980). Mands for verbalization. *Behavior Modification, 4*, 230–245

Matching-to-Sample. A language teaching strategy; a child's response is reinforced only if it matches a sample; helps generate rule-based responding based on physical or functional similarity.

Teaching matching-to-sample on the basis of physical similarity:

- Display an array of stimuli in front of the child (e.g., a book, a ball, and a pencil)
- Hold a sample and show it to the child (e.g., a different book than the one displayed in front of the child)
- Ask the child to match it to the one displayed
- Reinforce the correct matching (e.g., pointing to the book)

Teaching matching-to-sample on the basis of functional similarity

- Display an array of stimuli in front of the child (e.g., a large blue sneaker, a small brown ball)
- Hold a sample that matches the function of one of the objects but the physical property of the other object displayed (e.g., a small brown shoe) and show it to the child
- Ask the child to match it to the one displayed
- Reinforce the correct matching (e.g., the blue sneaker)

Milieu Teaching. A collection of child language intervention procedures that emphasize natural, functional, conversational communicative contexts for teaching language; a naturalistic child language teaching method; uses natural consequences as reinforcers; includes the Mand-Model and Incidental Teaching Method (described earlier in this section).

Narrative Skills Training. A speaker's description of events (stories, episodes) and experiences in a logically consistent, cohesive, temporally sequenced manner; analyzed in terms of a Story Grammar (described later in this section); an advanced language skill targeted during the final stages of intervention.

- Use the Event Structure (described earlier in this section) approach to give children experience in establishing Scripts (schemes of events)
  - play such scripts as grocery shopping, eating in a restaurant, birthday parties, camping trips, vacations, playing certain games, and so forth
  - play daily routine scripts (get children involved in daily activities)
  - repeatedly read or tell the same stories so the children memorize the words, temporal sequences, characters, and events
  - let the children act out the stories
  - let the children switch the roles on repeated scripts
- Ask children to narrate experiences as they play out scripts and assume different roles
- As you retell stories, pause before important phrases or critical descriptions so the children supply them
- Prompt the phrases and descriptions as the children hesitate; fade the prompts
- Ask the children to tell the stories or narrate events without enacting the scripts but with the help of pictures or slides
- Ask the children to tell stories or narrate events without scripts, pictures, or slides
- Ask the children to narrate new events or experiences (not rehearsed or scripted)

Nelson, N. W. (1993). *Childhood language disorders in context.* New York: Merrill.

Paul, R. (1995). *Language disorders from infancy through adolescence.* St. Louis, MO: C. V. Mosby.

Ripich, D. N., & Creaghead, N. A. (1994). *School discourse problems* (2nd ed.). San Diego, CA: Singular Publishing Group.

Naturalistic Child Language Teaching Method. An approach which emphasizes natural, functional, conversational communicative contexts for teaching language to children; uses loose training structure; uses natural consequences as reinforcers; includes Incidental

Teaching Method, Joint Action Routines or Interactions, Mand-Model, and Script Therapy (all described in this section).

Parallel-Talk. Describing or commenting upon what the child is doing during play activities; part of Indirect Language Stimulation.

- Arrange play activities designed to enhance opportunities for language production
- Play with the child
- Describe the child's actions (e.g., "you are playing with the ball, you are bouncing the ball")

Peer Modeling. A child language intervention method in which the peers are trained to model the target skills for the child.

- Select a peer who agrees to help and is acceptable to the client
- Have the peer observe your treatment sessions
- Describe the target behaviors, modeling and imitation sequence, and reinforcement procedures
- Let the peer model and reinforce the child's productions in your presence
- Refine the peer's skills in modeling the target behaviors
- Ask the peer to submit recorded language samples that document appropriate modeling outside the clinic
- Periodically assess the results of peer modeling and provide additional training to the peer

Reauditorization. Clinician's repetition of what a child says during language stimulation; often combined with such other techniques as modeling (often without requiring imitation); need more evidence to show its usefulness or effectiveness.

- Repeatedly model a target language feature in varied linguistic contexts (e.g., you say "the book is *on* the table; the cat is *on* the tree; the dog is *on* the house")
- Point to a target stimulus or ask a question (point to a bird on a tree; or ask "Where is the bird?"

- Repeat the child's production "in tree" or "bird is in the tree"

Recast. Expansion of a child's utterance type (sometimes presumed) into a different type of sentence; a method of play-oriented, unstructured, Indirect Language Stimulation.

- Arrange play activity designed to enhance opportunities for language production
- Play with the child
- Expand the child's utterance into a sentence type that may be different from the child's presumably intended sentence type (e.g., the child says "Big ball;" you expand it into a negative sentence, "No, it is not a big ball;" or expand it into a question form, "Is this a big ball?")
- Do not ask the child to imitate your recast sentences

Request for Repair. A listener's (clinician's in intervention sessions) use of various devices to let the client know that his or her expression was not clear and that the message needs to be altered.

- Ask the speaker (the child) to repeat
- Ask a question ("What do you mean?")
- Use negation to prompt the child to clarify a statement ("You did not have seventy friends at your birthday party, did you?")
- Model the correct response by saying what the child meant ("You mean you had seven friends at your birthday party").
- Turn a child's utterance into a question with a rising intonation ("You had seventy friends?")

Scaffolding. A collection of procedures to make it easier for a child to produce specific language behaviors or perform academic tasks; communicative assistance or support given to the child by peers and adults; a shared learning environment which promotes communication between the child and adults; ways to simplify communicative and academic tasks for the child.

To teach language use:

- Support the child in his or her attempts to speak
- Direct the child's attention to important aspects of learning and communication
- Give feedback to the child's questions and comments
- Give semantically contingent feedback
- Provide prompts and models
- Let peers help the child
- Encourage the child to ask questions
- Let the child take part in problem solving activities
- Expand and elaborate the child's utterances
- Fade the degree of support

To promote academic learning in a collaborative model:

- Ask the teacher to reduce academic demands that the child cannot meet or give more time for assignments
- Highlight important terms, issues, questions, definitions in a child's textbook; ask the child to find the meanings of terms in a dictionary
- Work on listening, reading, writing, and other skills that are required in the classroom

Kirchner, D. (1991). Reciprocal book reading. A discourse-based intervention strategy for the child with atypical language development. In T. Gallagher (Ed.), *Pragmatics of language: Clinical practice issues* (pp 307–332). San Diego, CA: Singular Publishing Group.

Paul, R. (1995). *Language disorders from infancy through adolescence*. St. Louis, MO: C. V. Mosby.

Ripich, D. N., & Creaghead, N. A. (1994). *School discourse problems* (2nd ed.). San Diego, CA: Singular Publishing Group.

Script Therapy. Language intervention procedure in which events and routines known to the child or made familiar by the clinician (Scripts) are used; procedures are similar to those under Event Structures and Joint Action Routines or Interactions (described earlier in this section); used in teaching advanced language skills including narrative skills; a script is usually not a written document although it may be in treatment; refers mostly to presumed ideas or a mental scheme a child may have about such common experiences as eating in a restaurant or grocery shopping.

- Select language targets appropriate for the children to be taught (e.g., such action-object-locative constructions as "Put the doll in the box")
- Select routinized scripts for each target (e.g., scattered toys that the mother and the child sort and put away before bed time)
- Assign different roles to the participants; assign one to yourself (e.g., one plays the role of the mother of a child being taught)
- Scatter several toys and have a box, a shelf, a table, and other objects for storing the toys
- Begin by saying something to initiate the script (routine activity) (e.g., "OK, it is bedtime! Let us pick these toys and put them away")
- Model target responses ("I am putting the doll in the box") and if the child imitates, reinforce
- Ask questions (e.g., "What are you doing?") and reinforce correct responses ("I am putting the car on the shelf")
- Complete the script and reenact the same or similar scripts
- Probe for generalized production (probe the same target responses with different scripts)

Paul, R. (1995). *Language disorders from infancy through adolescence.* St. Louis, MO: C. V. Mosby.

Young, K. T., & Lombardino, L. J. (1991). The efficacy of script contexts in language comprehension intervention with children who have mental retardation. *Journal of Speech and Hearing Research. 34*, 845–857.

Self-Talk. Clinician's description of her own activity as she plays with the child; a method of play-oriented, more or less structured, Indirect Language Stimulation.

- Arrange play activities designed to enhance opportunities for language production

- Play with the child
- Describe your own actions using language structures appropriate for the child (e.g., "I'm squeezing the rubber ducky here, see I'm squeezing.")

Story Grammar. The structure of narratives which may be a treatment target for children with language disorders; a story grammar includes the following elements:

- Setting statements (e.g., introduction to the story, the characters, the physical setting, the temporal context)
- Initiating events (e.g., episodes that begin a story)
- Internal response (e.g., the characters' emotions, reactions, thoughts)
- Internal plans (e.g., the characters' strategies for achieving their objectives)
- Attempts (e.g., actions the characters take to achieve their objectives)
- Direct consequences (e.g., results of actions)
- Reactions (e.g., the characters' response to the results)

Stein, N., & Glenn, C. (1979). An analysis of story comprehension in elementary school children. In R. Freedle (Ed.), *New directions in discourse processing* (Vol. 2, pp. 53–120). Norwood, NJ: Ablex.

Topic Initiation (Treatment for). The skill to start conversation with a new topic; a conversational skill; a pragmatic feature of language; a language treatment target; children with language disorders either fail to initiate topics or introduce inappropriate topics.

- Arrange a variety of stimuli that could trigger a new topic; objects, pictures, storybooks, topic cards (for children who can read), toys, structured play situations such as a kitchen and so forth
- Introduce one of the stimulus items or situations and draw the child's attention to it (e.g., a picture of a family setting up a tent in a park)

- Wait for the child to initiate conversation about the picture and the story
- If the child does not initiate a topic, instruct the child to say something about the picture
- If the child does not initiate, prompt it by beginning the story ("they are setting up a . . .)
- Lavishly praise the child for saying anything related to the topic depicted
- Accept statements that are remotely connected to the topic at hand; gradually, demand more relevant responses
- Do not interrupt the child or overly correct the forms of responses
- Ask the child to use the topic cards to initiate new topics
- Ask the child to think of new topics to talk about
- Prompt new topics
- Withdraw or fade such prompts, cues, cards, pictures and other special stimuli to make topic initiation more spontaneous
- Train parents to use your techniques so they can continue intervention at home

Topic Maintenance (Treatment for). A pragmatic language skill and treatment target; talking about a single general topic for extended duration; frequent and abrupt switching of conversational topics suggests lack of this skill.

- Target topic maintenance when training has moved to the conversational speech stage or sooner if the session structures allow it
- Let the child select topics of interest for talking
- Set a realistic duration for which you want the child to talk on a single topic; or set a target number of words to be produced on a topic
- Increase the duration or the number of target words in gradual steps

- Use such devices as *Tell me more. What about that? What happened next? Who said what? Where was it? When did that happen?* and so forth to stimulate more speech on the same topic
- Reinforce the child for maintaining the topic
- Stop the child when he or she abruptly switches the topic
- Move the child back to the target topic
- Train on a few topics and then probe with untrained topics to see if the skills have generalized
- Train on additional topic exemplars if the skills have not generalized

Turn Taking (Treatment for). Appropriate exchange of speaker and listener roles during conversation; a pragmatic language skill; an advanced treatment target; interrupting a speaker and not responding to cues to talk are indicators of deficient turn taking.

- Select turn taking as a target when treatment has advanced to conversational speech or sooner if the child can handle it
- Baserate the number of interruptions and failure to take cues to talk
- Design a signal for the child to talk (e.g., such verbal cues as "Your turn" or non-verbal cues as a hand gesture to suggest *you speak*)
- Design a signal that says *do not interrupt* or *do not talk* because it is your (clinician's) turn to talk (e.g., finger on your lips)
- Use such other discriminative stimuli as a real or toy microphone that you exchange with the child; the one holding the microphone talks and the other listens
- Reinforce the child for talking only when signaled or while holding the microphone
- Follow the same rule that you impose on the child (e.g., talk only when you hold the microphone)

- Teach the child to say "it is your turn"
- Reinforce the child for yielding the floor
- Teach turn taking until the child meets a performance criterion (e.g., no errors of turn taking in two consecutive conversational exchanges)
- Fade the signals or other special discriminative stimuli used to prompt the child
- Probe without signals or special discriminative stimuli
- Train until a probe criterion is met (at least 90% accuracy in turn taking while not receiving reinforcers)

Whole Language Approach. A philosophical approach to language, especially reading and writing, that has implications for oral language teaching; does not strictly refer to a method of teaching oral language; advocates that in teaching, language should not be broken down into components; believes that all aspects of literacy including reading, writing, listening, and talking should be simultaneously taught as an integrated whole; considers the Language-Based Classroom Model of intervention to be the best to teach language because all aspects of literacy can be effectively addressed; suggests that academic programs should be the basis of language teaching; advocates a naturalistic approach to language teaching; the approach needs efficacy research and specification and experimental evaluation of whole language teaching strategies.

- Select functional language skills that are based on the student's strength for intervention
- Include reading, writing, and speaking skills in your targets and integrate them with oral language training
- In the classroom setting, focus on developing language skills in language impaired children
- Conduct intervention in small or large groups (although some individual attention may be necessary in the beginning)

- Maintain the same theme across different days of training but vary the formats (stories, pictures, drawings, literature, dance)
- Introduce new concepts and ideas each day, but maintain the same theme for continuity
- Provide opportunities for the child to express verbally; assume the role of a facilitator, not instructor
- Promote child's active participation in therapy
- Elaborate and refine child's utterances
- Interact at the child's developmental level

Norris, J. A., & Damacio, J. S. (1990). Whole language in theory and practice: Implications for language intervention. *Language, Speech, and Hearing Services in Schools, 21*, 212–220.

Language Deviance in Children. Somewhat similar to the term Language Disorders in Children; includes a connotation of some abnormality in the acquisition or use of language for which there is little empirical support; not strictly a synonym for language disorders; treatment procedures the same as those for Language Disorders in Children.

Language Impairment. Generally the same as language disorders; includes an acceptable connotation of a disturbed function; may be used interchangeably with language disorder; treatment procedures the same as those for Language Disorders in Children.

Language-Learning Disorders. Generally the same as language disorders; links language disorder to a general learning disorder that negatively affects academic learning; often used in special educational contexts; treatment procedures the same as those for Language Disorders in Children.

Language Problems. Generally the same as language disorders; a more general term that may be used interchangeably with language disorders; treatment procedures the same as those for Language Disorders in Children.

Language Stimulation by Parents. Activities parents implement at home to stimulate language in infants and toddlers; may be the only recommendation for a child; may supplement or parallel clinicians' treatment.

- Assess the child and his or her family
- Assess the parents' education, sophistication, time commitment, and motivation to conduct regular activities at home
- Design a language stimulation program for the child
- Test the program in the clinic for a few sessions to make sure it works
- Have parents observe your sessions
- Train parents in the effective methods; model the methods frequently
- Have parents conduct a session or two in the clinic
- Give feedback and refine their skills
- Train them to keep records of therapy that you can evaluate
- Give parents simple, clear written instructions
- Give parents video taped samples of treatment techniques
- Periodically assess the child and the parents' sessions at home
- Suggest needed modifications and movement to higher levels of training
- Initiate formal treatment when your assessment indicates a need for it

Laryngeal Hyperkeratosis. A thickening of the laryngeal mucosa resulting from an abnormal growth of the epithelium; causes may include cigarette smoking, heavy alcohol use, environmental pollutants, dust, noxious gases, and strained and tense speaking habits; usually occurs on the true vocal folds; may sometimes be premalignant; voice treatment may include reduced exposure to the listed causal factors.

Laryngeal Leukoplakia. Appearance of white patches on the laryngeal mucosa; voice may be hoarse; may be premalignant; reduction in or elimination of smoking is recommended.

Laryngeal Stoma. An opening made into the trachea between the thyroid glands to allow for breathing in patients with laryngectomy.

Laryngeal Web. Growth of a thin membrane across portions of the vocal folds; may be congenital or induced by trauma later in life; negatively affects respiration; treatment is surgical removal.

Laryngectomee. A person who has had a partial or total Laryngectomy.

Laryngectomy. Surgical removal of all or part of the larynx because of disease or trauma.

Treatment Procedures, Laryngectomy

Preoperative Evaluation and Counseling

- Work as a member of the rehabilitation team
- In consultation with the surgeon, counsel the patient and the family about the effects of medical treatment on communication
- Invite and answer all questions from the patient and the family members; give answers that are consistent with advice from other professionals on the team
- Do not withhold information if the patient would like to hear it
- Obtain a sample of the patient's speech and writing; make an assessment of client's communication skills
- Describe various methods of speaking without a larynx; discuss communication options that may be preferable to the client; be consistent with the surgeon's preferences and recommendations
- Reassure the patient that he or she will talk again by using new techniques
- Have the patient meet and speak with a rehabilitated Laryngectomee who has mastered Alaryngeal Speech

Postoperative Management

- If no prior counseling, discuss the current condition of the patient and the prospects for new methods of communication
- Review the information provided during the preoperative counseling

- Discuss methods of Alaryngeal Speech (described later in this section)
- Demonstrate how electronic speech aids work
- Teach the patient to use a Pneumatic Device for Alaryngeal Speech (described later in this section), if appropriate, to support immediate communication
- Discuss the patient's rehabilitation plan; be cautious in making prognostic statements
- Give written information on rehabilitation plans and possibilities for the patient to read later
- Arrange a visit from a rehabilitated Laryngectomee to encourage the patient

Teaching New Methods of Communication

General Principles

- Select an appropriate method of communication that the client prefers, judged to be efficient, and is practical
- Teach the client to use the new method of communication
- Select either a Pneumatic Device for Alaryngeal Speech or an Electronic Device for Alaryngeal Speech (both described later in this section) for permanent communication
- Let the client use a pneumatic device during the early postsurgical period as it is easier to use within days after surgery; let the client switch to an electronic device if that is preferred
- Begin to teach the use of an electronic device only after the neck and throat areas recover from swelling and tenderness and the surgical suture lines heal
- Teach tracheoesophageal speech if the patient is surgically prepared for it
- Consider both individual and group therapy sessions
- Determine the frequency of treatment sessions based on the patient's physical condition
- Consider daily sessions in the beginning if the patient's physical stamina permits them
- Hold at least one weekly session
- Get family members involved in training sessions

- Let the patient's performance and progress dictate the pace of therapy
- Ask the client to practice the new method of communication at home

Teach Alaryngeal Speech with Electronic Devices

- Select a neck-held electronic larynx after discussing various models with the patient
- Demonstrate first what the instrument sounds like and then how speech produced with its help sounds like
- Experiment with the best position on the neck (usually under the jaw); let the head of the device make good contact with the skin without pressing it
- Manipulate the button for sound production and ask the patient to count aloud
- Ask the patient to clearly shape the words with the mouth
- Ask the patient not to exhale forcefully
- Teach the patient to handle the device
- Instruct the patient to coordinate sound and speech and to turn off the sound when not talking
- Reduce the patient's rate of speech to increase intelligibility
- Teach the patient to increase articulatory precision by practicing words that begin with voiceless consonants
- Shape progressively longer utterances
- Teach the client to maintain eye contact with the listener

Teach Alaryngeal Speech with Pneumatic devices

- Use pneumatic devices during the early phase of rehabilitation
- Select a pneumatic device after discussing various options
- Teach the patient to place the cup end of the device firmly over the <u>Laryngeal Stoma</u> so that there is no air leak
- Ask the patient to hold the cup end over the stoma and produce a sound by blowing out

- Ask the patient to blow out two and three sounds for every breath
- Ask the patient to change the pitch by increasing the air pressure
- Ask the patient to place the mouth piece on top of the tongue, while keeping the cup end over the Laryngeal Stoma
- Ask the patient to say vowels and then words
- Shape progressively longer utterances
- Give appropriate positive and corrective feedback

Teach Esophageal Speech

- Begin esophageal speech training soon after patient starts eating food orally
- Describe the anatomy and the physiology of esophageal speech production
- Describe esophageal sound production to the patient
- Use diagrams to explain esophageal speech
- Teach the client the production of esophageal sound
- Try various procedures and settle on the one most effective with the client
- Teach the patient to use the injection method of taking air into the esophagus
    - ask the patient to press the tongue tip against the alveolar ridge to push the air back toward esophagus without the tongue making contact with the pharyngeal wall (glossal press)
    - ask the client to press the tongue tip against the alveolar ridge and to move the tongue back to make contact with the pharyngeal wall; thus push air back into the esophagus (glossopharyngeal press)
    - ask the patient to keep the velopharyngeal port closed
    - ask the client to inject the air in an audible manner, producing the sound called the "klunk"
- Teach the patient to use the inhalation method of taking air into the esophagus if necessary; be aware that some experts use only the injection method for most of their patients

- teach the patient to synchronize the air intake through the stoma with air intake through the mouth into the upper esophagus; relaxed PE segment and the resulting negative pressure there will help air movement into upper esophagus
- Ask the patient to produce plosive consonants to stimulate esophageal sound
- Instruct the patient to say ta-ta-ta
- Ask the patient to use easy injection of air and say a series of ta-ta-ta
- Reinforce a likely emergence of esophageal sound
- Teach the patient to puff the cheeks out and move the air trapped in the mouth from one side to another; instruct the patient to move this trapped air quickly into the esophagus
- Ask the patient to produce words that typically trigger sound production: *church, stop, skate, scotch*, and *scratch*
- Use single phonemes initially
- Move on to single syllable words
- Increase response complexity
- Ask the patient to slow down the rate of speech

Teach Tracheoesophageal Speech

- Select a Voice Prosthesis for a patient who has undergone Tracheoesophageal Fistulization/Puncture)
- Insert the voice prosthesis into the fistula; make sure the fistula is properly healed; also make sure that there is no leakage of fluid around or through the prosthesis
- Ask the patient to inhale, occlude the stoma with a finger, and exhale
- Ask the client to produce sound as the air from the lungs enters the P-E Segment through the voice prostheses
- Have the patient practice sound production
- Shape the sound into speech
- Increase the length of utterances
- Give appropriate feedback

Andrews, M. L. (1995). *Manual of voice treatment: Pediatrics to geriatrics*. San Diego, CA: Singular Publishing Group.

Casper, J. K., & Colton, R. H. (1993). *Clinical manual for laryngectomy and head and neck cancer rehabilitation.* San Diego, CA: Singular Publishing Group.

Laryngitis. Irritated and swollen vocal folds; causes include vocally abusive behaviors and infection.

Laryngitis, Chronic. Irritated and swollen vocal folds of long history; Hoarseness is the primary result; lowered vocal pitch and vocal tiredness also may result; may lead to vocal nodules or polyps.

- Impose vocal rest without whispering
- Reduce vocally abusive behaviors

Laryngitis, Traumatic. Irritated and swollen vocal folds; result of such vocally abusive behaviors as shouting, screaming, and loud cheering; hoarseness is the primary result.

- Do not recommend voice treatment for such temporary laryngitis as that following enthusiastic participation in ball games; natural period rest (one night's sleep) may be adequate
- Reduce vocally abusive behaviors if they persist

Laryngoplasty. Surgical treatment to improve phonation in people with vocal cord paralysis or weakness; involves medial displacement of vocal cords with the help of implant materials to promote better approximation.

Left-Hand Manual Alphabet. A manual communication method developed by L. Chen for clients with right hand paralysis; appropriate for some clients with aphasia; the signs closely approximate the letters; used in teaching Augmentative Communication-Gestural (unaided).

Chen, L. Y. (1971). Manual communication by combined alphabet and gestures. *Archives of Physical Medicine and Rehabilitation, 52,* 381–384.

Lesson Plan. A brief treatment plan which describes short-term goals and procedures; in case of student clinicians, approved by the clinical supervisor.

- Use Operational Definitions in writing treatment goals
- Give clear and brief description of procedures to be used

Logical Validity. Consistency of statements that do not violate rules of logic; treatment procedures that may be logically consistent; no assurance that the procedures have experimental support; contrasted with Empirical Validity.

Maintenance Strategy. Methods designed to promote the production of treated communicative skills in natural environments and sustained over time; to be planned from the beginning of treatment; requires the extension of treatment to natural settings and training the client's significant others to help evoke and reinforce the target skills; all aspects of treatment including stimulus variables, response characteristics, and response consequences should be manipulated to achieve maintenance.

Stimulus Manipulations

- Select common, functional, client-specific stimulus items, preferably objects; let the client bring stimuli from home (e.g., a girl could bring her toys to serve as stimuli in speech or language training)
- Select colorful, unambiguous, and realistic pictures
- Select simple and common verbal stimuli that are used to evoke the target responses
- Vary the audience; have family members and other persons participate as conversational partners in treatment sessions
- Vary physical setting controls; conduct informal treatment outside the clinic room, in cafeterias, campus walks, library, bookstore, home, and other natural settings.

Response Considerations

- Select client-specific and functional responses for treatment targets
- Train multiple exemplars of each target skill and at each level of response complexity
- Take training to complex levels of target skills: always end treatment with sufficient training at the conversational level

Contingency Manipulation

- Use intermittent reinforcement schedules in the latter stages of training
- Use conditioned reinforcers (tokens with back-up reinforcers)
- Delay reinforcement in the latter stages of training
- Let the family members and others watch treatment sessions so they can better understand the treatment targets and teaching methods

- Train significant others in evoking and prompting the target behaviors at home and other nonclinical settings
- Train significant others in reinforcing the production of target behaviors at home and other nonclinical settings
- Reinforce generalized responses; have parents and others reinforce generalized productions at home
- Teach Reinforcement Priming to the client (e.g., teach the client to draw attention to his or her production of target behaviors at home so the ignoring parents can pay attention and reinforce the client)
- Hold informal Training Sessions In Natural Environments
- Teach Self-Control (Self-Monitoring) Procedures (e.g., counting one's target behaviors)
- Give treatment for a sufficient duration
- Follow-Up and arrange for Booster Treatment

Management of Behavioral Contingencies. A clinician's or a parent's skill in arranging effective stimuli for target communication skills, requiring the production of specified skills, and in promptly and effectively providing differential feedback for the correct and incorrect productions; inherent to all behavioral intervention techniques.

- Provide effective stimuli for target behaviors; use pictures, objects, enacted events, instructions, demonstrations, models, prompts, manual guidance, visual and tactile cues, and other stimuli for the target behavior
- Specify the response form; demonstrate what the client is expected to produce
- Give feedback promptly, clearly, naturally, and as frequently as needed

Mand-Model. A child language intervention method which uses components of Incidental Teaching Method; uses typical adult-child interactions in a play-oriented setting to teach functional communication skills; for procedures, see Language Disorders in Children; Treatment of Language Disorders: Specific Techniques or Programs.

Mands. A class of verbal behaviors that are triggered by a state of motivation; includes requests, commands, and demands; need to create a state of motivation to teach mands; often reinforced with primary reinforcers.

- Create a state of motivation:
  - arrange treatment around lunch or breakfast time so food may be used as a reinforcer (hunger is the state of motivation)
  - hold food in front of the child until the child asks for it
  - place attractive toys on a high shelf and give them to the child only when requested
  - offer a food item the child does not like (the child should verbally refuse it)
  - eat something the child is fond of without offering it (the child should request it)
  - give a tightly closed jar with candy in it (the child should ask you to open it)
- Reinforce promptly with the displayed or held back item; remove promptly an aversive item presented when the child makes an appropriate response

Manual Shorthand. A method of communication that combines the Left-Hand Manual Alphabet with gestures; expressed by left-hand gestures; appropriate for clients with right-hand paralysis; used in teaching Augmentative Communication-Gestural (Unaided).

Chen, L. Y. (1971). Manual communication by combined alphabet and gestures. *Archives of Physical Medicine and Rehabilitation, 52*, 381–384.

Manual Guidance. Physical guidance provided to shape a response; the Phonetic Placement Method is similar to manual guidance; needed when the client cannot imitate a response.

- Use your fingers to shape articulators
- Take the client's hand and make it touch the target picture while training comprehension of commands
- Use tongue depressors to move the tongue to desired positions

- Apply slight digital pressure to the laryngeal area to lower a client's pitch
- Apply a slight pressure on the chin of a child who does not readily open the mouth

Matching. A method in which subjects of similar characteristics are placed in the experimental and control groups used to evaluate treatment effects; part of the Group Design Strategy.

- Find pairs of subjects with the same or similar characteristics (age, gender, severity of the disorder, socioeconomic status)
- Assign one of the pair to the experimental group and the other to the control group
- Match groups on the basis of group means if pair-wise matching is not possible (the two groups with the same average IQ, for instance)

Mechanical Corrective Feedback. A method to reduce incorrect responses in treatment; also known as Biofeedback; feedback is presented soon after an incorrect response is made; includes such feedback as provided on a computer monitor for incorrect responses (e.g., undesirable vocal pitch or intensity) and electromyographic feedback on muscle tension.

Meninges. Membranes that cover the brain.

Mental Retardation. Intellectual, social, and adaptive behaviors that are significantly below normal during the developmental period which extends up to age 18; communicative problems are a significant aspect of retardation; mostly, the treatment procedures for Language Disorders in Children are applicable with the following special considerations:

- Recommend or initiate treatment as early as possible
- Get the family involved in early Language Stimulation
- Get the help of other specialists including special educators and psychologists

- Consider the academic or occupational demands made on the client; select targets that help meet those demands
- Sequence the target behaviors carefully; use small step increments
- Use objects and events more than pictures as treatment stimuli
- Train in varied naturalistic settings to promote generalized production
- Use primary reinforcers initially and fade them
- Shape language behaviors in successive stages
- Use modeling frequently and then fade it
- Implement a systematic maintenance program
- Follow-up and arrange for booster treatment

Metronome-Paced Speech. A method used to slow down the rate of speech; the client is asked to pace a syllable or a word to each beat of a metronome; used in the treatment of stuttering and cluttering; see also Stuttering, Treatment; Treatment of Stuttering: Specific Techniques or Programs.

- Begin treatment with a slow beat that reduces the rate of speech to a level where stuttering or cluttering is markedly reduced or eliminated
- Have the client practice slow speech until fluency is stabilized
- Fade the metronome by gradually increasing the rate of its beat until the speech rate and prosody approximate the normal

Mixed Dysarthrias. A type of motor speech disorder that is a combination of two or more pure dysarthrias; the neuropathology is varied depending on the types of dysarthrias that are mixed; frequent causes include multiple strokes or multiple neurological diseases; speech disorders are varied and dependent on the types of pure dysarthrias that are mixed; select appropriate treatment targets and procedures described under Dysarthria, Treatment; in addition, consider the following that apply especially to mixed dysarthrias:

- Make a thorough assessment of the client's symptom complex of mixed dysarthria
- Identify the dominant type, if any, and describe the major speech problems
- Select speech targets that when treated will immediately improve communication
- Treat those targets like you would in the case of pure dysarthrias

Duffy, J. R. (1995). *Motor speech disorders*. St. Louis, MO: C. V. Mosby.

Johns, D. F. (Ed.). (1985). *Clinical management of neurogenic communicative disorders*. Boston: Little, Brown

Yorkston, K. M., Beukelman, D. R., & Bell, K. R. (1988). *Clinical management of dysarthric speakers*. Austin, TX: Pro-Ed.

Mode (of response). Manner or method of a response; includes imitation, oral reading, and conversational speech.

Modeling. Clinician's production of a target behavior for the client to imitate; needed when the clinician cannot evoke a response; used frequently in treating communicative disorders.

- Provide live or mechanically delivered model (audio or video taped or computer-presented)
- Use the client's own correct response as a model (presented mechanically)
- Model frequently in the beginning stages of treatment
- Ask the client to imitate as closely as possible
- Reinforce the client for correct imitations or approximations
- Withdraw or fade modeling in gradual steps as the client's imitative responses stabilize

Modeled Trial. An opportunity to imitate a response when the clinician models it.

- Place stimulus item in front of the client; show an object, or demonstrate an action
- Ask the predetermined question (e.g., "What is this?")
- Immediately model correct response ("Johnny, say...")
- Wait a few seconds for the client to respond

- Consequate the response if it is a modeled training trial
- Do not consequate the response if it is a modeled baseline trial
- Record the response on the recording sheet
- Remove stimulus item
- Wait 2–3 seconds to signify end of trial

Hegde, M. N. (1993). *Treatment procedures in communicative disorders* (2nd ed.). Austin, TX: Pro-Ed.

Modification of Treatment Procedures. See Treatment of Communicative Disorders: Procedural Modifications.

Monterey Fluency Program. A treatment program for adults and children who stutter; behaviorally based; a fluency shaping program; for procedures see Stuttering, Treatment; Treatment of Stuttering: Specific Techniques or Programs.

Moto-Kinesthetic Method. An articulation treatment method developed by Young and Stinchfield-Hawk; is similar to Phonetic Placement Method; emphasizes awareness of kinesthetic movement involved in articulation; to be used in the initial stages of treatment; clinician manipulates client's articulators with her hand to promote kinesthetic awareness.

Motor Speech Disorders. A group of speech disorders associated with neuropathology affecting the motor control of speech muscles or motor programming of speech movements; include Dysarthria and Apraxia of Speech.

Multiple Baseline Design. A set of single-subject designs in which the effects of treatment are demonstrated by showing that untreated baselines did not change and that only the treated baselines did; useful in integrating treatment research with service delivery; has three variations: across behaviors, settings, and subjects.

Multiple baseline across behaviors design. A single subject design in which several behaviors are sequentially taught to show that only treated behavior changed and hence the treatment was effective.

- Select three or more target behaviors
- Establish baselines on all selected target behaviors
- Teach the first behavior to a Training Criterion
- Repeat baselines on the remaining untreated behaviors
- Teach the next behavior and repeat the baselines on the remaining untreated behaviors
- Continue to alternate baselines and treatment until all the behaviors are trained

Multiple baseline across settings design. A single-subject design in which a behavior is sequentially taught in different settings to show that the behavior changed only in a treated setting and hence the treatment was effective.

- Baserate a target behavior in three or more settings (e.g., clinic, home, school, or office)
- Teach the behavior in one setting
- Repeat the baserates in the remaining untreated settings
- Teach the behavior in another setting
- Continue to alternate baserates and teaching in different settings until the behavior is trained in all settings

Multiple baselines across subjects design. A single-subject research design in which several subjects are taught a behavior sequentially to show that only treated subjects changed and hence treatment was effective.

- Select a target behavior that needs to be taught to three or more clients
- Baserate the target behaviors in all subjects
- Treat one of the subjects
- Repeat the baserates on the untreated subjects
- Treat the second subject
- Repeat the baserates on untreated subjects
- Alternate treatment and baserates until all the clients are trained

Hegde, M. N. (1994). *Clinical research in communicative disorders* (2nd ed.). Austin, TX: Pro-Ed.

Multiple Causation. The philosophical position that most events, including communicative behaviors and their disorders, have several causes.

Mutational Falsetto. Continuation of prepubertal voice after attaining puberty; voice is high-pitched.

- Have medical conformation of laryngeal maturation
- Establish a lower pitched voice; use techniques described under Voice Disorders; Treatment of Disorders of Loudness and Pitch.

Narrative Skills. A language skill in describing events in a sequential, chronologically correct, and logically consistent manner; treatment procedures described under Language Disorders in Children; Treatment of Language Disorders: Specific Techniques or Programs; Narrative Skills Training.

Nasendoscope. A mechanical device used to examine internal organs illuminated by a fiberoptic tube inserted through the nose.

Nativism. A philosophical position that humans are born with certain forms of knowledge that they need not learn through experience; basis for nativists' assertion that children are born with knowledge of universal grammar, sentence structure, or phonological rules.

Natural Settings. Nonclinical settings where clients communicate for the most part; communication in such settings is always a final treatment target; in the case of infants and toddlers, treatment may be implemented in such settings; extending treatment to such settings is essential to promote response maintenance.

Natural-Sounding Fluency. A stuttering treatment target when such techniques as Delayed Auditory Feedback, Metronome-Paced Speech, and Rate Reduction are used; see Stuttering, Treatment; Treatment of Stuttering: Specific Techniques or Programs for additional information.

- Fade explicit management of airflow
- Fade the use of metronome
- Fade the use of delayed auditory feedback
- Increase the rate of speech to near-normal levels
- Teach variations in intonation
- Teach normal rhythm of speech

Neck Brace. A brace around the neck used to stabilize the weakened neck muscles; often used in treating clients with dysarthrias.

Negative Reinforcers. Aversive events that are removed, reduced, postponed, or prevented; responses that accomplish these increase in frequency; less useful than positive reinforcers in teaching communicative skills.

Neural Anastomosis. Connecting a branch of an undamaged nerve to a damaged nerve; a surgical treatment for certain dysarthric clients; a branch of the intact XIIth cranial nerve may be connected to the damaged VIIth cranial nerve to restore function and appearance.

Neuritic Plaques. Clumps of degenerating neurons; present in the brains of Alzheimer's patients and some normal elderly persons.

Neurofibrillary Tangles. Twisted and tangled neurofibrils; a basic neuropathology of Alzheimer's Disease.

Neurogenic Fluency Disorders. Somewhat varied problems of fluency that have a demonstrated neurological basis; also known as neurogenic stuttering; may follow a stroke, head trauma, extrapyramidal diseases, tumor, dementia, and drugs prescribed for asthma and depression; to be distinguished from stuttering which is developmental with no gross neuropathology; may be persistent or transient; little or no research on treatment effects and efficacy; suggested techniques based on reported clinical experiences; evaluate the results of selected procedures carefully; abandon procedures that do not produce results with given clients.

- Make a thorough assessment and document neurological basis for the fluency disorder
- Reduce the speech rate to reduce or eliminate dysfluencies
- Use a Pacing Board to help the client reduce the speech rate
- Experiment with Delayed Auditory Feedback (DAF) to see if it is effective in slowing the speech rate
- Experiment with auditory masking to see if it is helpful
- Be aware that clients who exhibit stuttering along with slow and effortful speech may not benefit from pacing devices, DAF, and masking

- Consider relaxation and biofeedback to reduce speech muscle tension; evaluate the results carefully

Helm-Estabrooks, N. (1986). Diagnosis and management of neurogenic stuttering. In K. O. St. Louis, (Ed.). *The atypical stutterer* (pp. 193–217). New York: Academic Press.

Rosenbek, J. C. (1984). Stuttering secondary to nervous damage. In R. F. Curlee & W. H. Perkins (Eds.), *Nature and treatment of stuttering* (pp. 31–48). Austin, TX: Pro-Ed.

Nonexclusion Time-Out. Response-contingent arrangement of a brief duration of time in which all interaction is terminated; the client is not removed from the setting; one of the Direct Methods of Response Reduction; often used in communication training.

- Give response contingent signal to start time-out (e.g., saying, "Stop" as soon as a dysfluency occurs); do not let the client talk during time-out
- Turn your face away from the client
- Stay motionless for 5 seconds
- Turn toward the client, and continue the interaction

Noniconic Symbols. Abstract, geometric shapes that do not look like what they suggest; the meaning of such shapes to be established by training; more difficult to learn than Iconic Symbols, but more flexible; plastic chips or various shapes are an example; used in teaching Augmentative Communication, Gestural-Assisted (aided).

Nonpenetrating (Closed-Head) Injury. A head injury in which the skull may or may not be fractured or lacerated and the Meninges remain intact.

Non-SLIP (Non-Speech Language Initiation Program). A nonspeech communication program that uses the Premack-type, color-coded plastic shapes each associated with a word; developed and researched by Joseph Carrier, Jr.; the client learns to communicate by arranging them in sequence to form sentences; also used to promote oral language acquisition in initially minimally verbal children; used in teaching Augmentative Communication, Gestural-Assisted (aided).

Nonverbal Corrective Feedback. A method used to reduce incorrect responses in treatment; feedback is presented soon after an incorrect response is made; includes various forms of gestures, hand signals, and facial expressions; a form of Corrective Feedback; often paired with Verbal Corrective Feedback.

Normal Prosody. Normal or socially acceptable rhythm, stress, intonation (pitch variation), intensity, transition between words and phrases, correct phrasing and pausing at appropriate junctures, and acceptable rate of speech; a target in treating various disorders of communication including apraxia of speech, cluttering and stuttering, dysarthria, foreign accent reduction, hearing impairment, voice disorders, and so forth.

- Select a particular aspect of prosody for treatment (e.g., pitch variations)
- Model the target behavior
- Demonstrate the target on a computer screen, if possible
- Tape record the model and play it
- Ask the client to match the live or recorded model (imitate)
- Shape the target behavior in successive and progressively more complex steps
- Reinforce any movement in the direction of the model
- Set a higher level of response (e.g., sentences) when the target (a certain pitch or intensity) is achieved at a lower level (e.g., phrases)
- Give maximum feedback including auditory and visual feedback

Hargrove, P. M., & McGarr, N. S. (1994). *Prosody management of communication disorders*. San Diego, CA: Singular Publishing Group.

Normative Strategy. An approach to selecting target behaviors for clients based on age-based norms and developmental sequences; often used in selecting target speech sounds and language structures for children; some clinicians question its relevance and assumptions; contrasted with client-specific strategy.

- Assess the communicative behaviors of the child to determine potential treatment targets
- Select behaviors that the child should already have acquired based on the age-based norms
- Teach the selected behaviors in the normative sequence in which they are acquired

Norms. Average (mean) performance of a typical group of persons on a selected test in its standardization process; frequently established with the method of cross-sectional sampling of a group of children; most common problems are small sample size and limited sampling of behaviors measured; frequently used in selecting treatment targets.

Objectivity. Agreement among different observers who observe or measure the same event in the same manner; needed for treatment procedures so they can be replicated.

Omission training. Reinforcing a person for not exhibiting a certain behavior; the same as Differential Reinforcement of Other Behavior.

Open-Head Injury. The same as Penetrating Head Injury.

Operant Aggression. Aggressive behavior directed against the source of an aversive stimulus; a potential undesirable side-effect of punishment; contrasted with elicited aggression.

Operational Definitions. Definition of variables in measurable terms.

- Specify the topographic aspects of the target behavior (e.g., production of /s/ in word-initial positions, phrases, sentences)
- Specify the mode in which the response will be measured (e.g., reading, conversational speech)
- Specify the stimuli and settings (e.g., when shown pictures, in the clinic, or at home)
- Specify the accuracy criterion (e.g., 90% correct)

Overcorrection. A procedure used to reduce behaviors by requiring the person to eliminate the effects of his or her misbehavior (Restitution) and practice its counterpart, a desirable behavior (Positive Practice); both described under Imposition of Work.

Pacing Board. A wooden board that has a series of colored slots that are separated by ridges; used in reducing the speech rate of clients with motor speech disorders; the speaker touches one slot for each word spoken.

Paired-Stimuli Approach. An articulation treatment method; uses correct production of sounds in a Key Word to teach correct production of the same sounds misarticulated in other words; procedures described under Articulation and Phonological Disorders; Treatment of Articulation and Phonological Disorders: Specific Techniques or Programs.

Palate Reshaping Prosthesis. An intraoral device that lowers the palatal arch by artificially increasing its bulk; may be designed with teeth to replacing the missing teeth of the patient; helps the tongue with limited vertical movement to make contact with the hard palate to chew food.

Pantomime. A method of communication in which the speaker acts out a message by gestures and bodily movements; a target communication skill for some nonverbal or minimally verbal clients who can use gestures and bodily movements; unlike in other gestural systems, uses whole- as well as part-body movements; often more concrete and easier to understand than other gestures; used in teaching Augmentative Communication-Gestural (unaided).

Papillomas. Wart-like growths on the larynx; thought to be of viral origin; may be life-threatening if they block the airway; may be a recurring condition; treatment is laser surgery, which also needs to be repeated; may need voice therapy to make the best possible use of the compromised larynx.

- Teach the client to achieve appropriate pitch and loudness; use techniques described under Voice Disorders; Treatment of Disorders of Loudness and Pitch.
- Teach proper respiration control; treat any other voice symptom with Specific Normal Voice Facilitation Techniques (described under Voice Disorders)

Paradigm of Treatment. An overall philosophy or viewpoint of treatment.

Paraphasias. Unintended word or sound substitutions.

Paradoxical Effects. Increase in response rates when a known response reduction procedure is used; potential side-effect of punishment.

- Always watch for undesirable side-effects when using response reduction (punishment) procedures
- Terminate the punishment procedure when paradoxical effects are evident
- Always reinforce desirable target behaviors and minimize the use of response reduction procedures

Parallel Talk. A child language treatment method; describing or commenting upon what the child is doing during play activities; procedure described under Language Disorders in Children; Treatment of Language Disorders: Specific Techniques or Programs.

Parent Training. Preparing parents (or other family members) to conduct informal treatment at home; to conduct maintenance activities to sustain treatment gains at home and other natural settings; see Language Stimulation by Parents; Maintenance Strategy; Peer Training.

Parkinson's Disease. A progressive neurological syndrome associated with depigmentation of the substantia nigra, a midbrain structure functionally related to the basal ganglia; there is loss of ability to produce or store dopamine; symptoms include Tremor, Rigidity, depression, visuospatial disturbances, and Bradykinesia; irregular and less legible hand-writing; soft, monotonous, and rapid speech; crowded word productions without the usual pauses between phrases; general management procedures described under Dementia; in addition, consider the following suggestions:

- Reduce the rate of speech to increase intelligibility
- Use a Pacing Board

- Decrease monotonous tone of voice
- Increase vocal intensity (subject to improvement of chest musculature functioning)
- Increase pauses between phrases
- Monitor the changes (if any) that occur with specific medication (such as Levodopa (L-Dopa)

Partial Modeling. Withdrawing modeling of complete sentences in gradual steps; a method of Fading.
- Initially model complete sentences for the client to imitate (e.g., "The book is on the table")
- Drop the last word when it is time to fade modeling ("The book is on the . . .")
- Drop additional words, one word at a time, on subsequent trials ("The book is on . . .;" "The book is . . .;" "The book . . .," etc.)

P-E Segment. Pharyngeal-esophageal segment; a part of the pharynx and the esophagus; muscle fibers from the cricopharyngeus, esophagus, and inferior constrictor blend at this site to create a sphincter that can reduce the cross-sectional area of the esophagus.

Peer Modeling. A child language intervention method in which the peers are trained to model the target skills for the child client; procedure described under Language Disorders in Children; Treatment of Language Disorders: Specific Techniques or Programs.
- Select a peer who agrees to help and is acceptable to the client
- Have the peer observe your treatment sessions
- Describe the target behaviors, modeling and imitation sequence, and reinforcement procedures
- Let the peer model and reinforce the child's productions in your presence
- Refine the peer's skills in modeling the target behaviors
- Ask the peer to submit recorded language samples that document appropriate modeling outside the clinic

Periodically assess the results of peer modeling and provide additional training to the peer

Peer Training. Training peers of clients to evoke and reinforce target behaviors in natural settings; a Maintenance Strategy.

- Ask the peers to initially observe your treatment sessions
- Describe the target skills the client is being taught
- Let the peers count the occurrence of the skill along with you
- Give them feedback on their counting
- Train the peers to prompt, evoke, model, and reinforce the target communication skill
- Have them conduct a session in your presence
- Give them feedback and refine their skills
- Give them simple, clear written instructions
- Give them a sample of video tape of treatment procedures
- Ask them to monitor the target skills in natural settings
- Ask them to audio record a monitoring session outside the clinic or submit data recorded on paper
- Periodically review data submitted
- Periodically assess the client who is taught by the peers
- Initiate clinical treatment if peer training is not effective or their training cannot be improved

Penetrating (Open-Head) Injury. An injury where the skull is perforated or fractured and the Meninges are torn or lacerated.

Perceptual Training. The same as Auditory Discrimination Training; in articulation treatment, it is assumed that the clients should first learn to discriminate between speech sounds others produce before learning to produce them; in language treatment, it is assumed that the clients should comprehend language structures before learning to produce them; both assumptions questioned by some clinicians.

In articulation treatment:

- Present correct and incorrect productions of the target sounds alternatively

- Ask the child to judge each production as correct or incorrect
- Do not ask the child to produce the sounds
- Move to production training when the client can consistently discriminate your correct and incorrect presentations

In language treatment:

- Teach nonverbal responses to verbal stimuli
- Ask the child to show objects or pictures you name
- Ask the child to follow directions and commands
- Do not ask the child to produce oral language
- Move to production training of a given language structure when the client can comprehend the meaning of that structure when spoken

Peristalsis. Constricting and relaxing movements of a tubular structure (such as the pharynx) to move its contents (such as food in the pharynx); pharyngeal peristalsis may be disordered in patients with Dysphagia.

Perpetuation of Aversive Methods. Continued use of aversive (punishment) methods because of negative reinforcement received by those who use such methods.

Perseveration. Tendency to persist with the same response even though the stimulus has changed; often seen in patients with brain injury.

Phonetic Derivation. The use of Shaping procedures (progressive approximation) to teach correct articulation to clients who do not imitate the clinician's productions; the procedure involves breaking the target sound production into its simpler components, teaching them in sequence, and finally practicing the integrated response (e.g., teaching the production of /f/ by first gently biting on the lower lip and then adding other response components).

Phonetic Placement Method. An articulation treatment method; used when the client cannot imitate the modeled sound production; uses instruction, physical guidance, and visual feedback on how target sounds are produced;

often used as a component of a comprehensive treatment program.

- Describe how the target sound is produced
- Demonstrate how the sound is produced
- Show the placement of articulators
- Give maximum visual feedback; use a mirror and drawing of articulatory placements; use palatograms and breath indicators
- Show the differences between correct and incorrect productions of the same sound
- Help position the tongue of the client with tongue blades
- Use your fingers to manipulate and correctly position the client's articulators
- Let the client feel the presence and absence of laryngeal vibrations

Phonological Disorders. Multiple errors of articulation that form patterns based on Distinctive Features or Phonological Processes; the treatment target is to eliminate phonological processes.

Phonological Disorders (treatment of). See Articulation and Phonoloigcal Disorders.

Phonological Processes. Multiple ways in which children simplify adult production of speech sounds; these include such categories of processes as Deletion Processes, Substitution Processes, and Assimilation Processes; persistent processes in children are targets of intervention; treatment is directed against eliminating a phonological process; see Articulation and Phonological Disorders, Treatment of Articulation and Phonological Disorders: Specific Techniques or Programs.

Phrases (Word Combinations). Productions that contain two or more words; grammatically incomplete, hence not sentences; treatment targets for language impaired children.

- Teach a few First Words

- Create two-word phrases out of words the child already has learned (e.g., such nouns and adjectives as *big man* or *small box*)
- Teach them with either Indirect Language Stimulation or Direct Language Treatment Approaches

Physical Setting Generalization. Production of trained responses in a setting not used in training; an important clinical goal; measured on a Probe; typically not reinforced.
- Select stimuli for treatment targets from the client's home
- Use common stimuli found in nonclinical settings
- Give training in varied physical settings

Physical Stimulus Generalization. Production of trained responses in the presence of untrained stimuli because of their similarity to trained stimuli; an important treatment goal; typically measured on a Probe; usually not reinforced.
- Use varied stimuli in training
- Use stimuli from the client's home
- Prefer objects to pictures

Pic Symbols. A set of Pictogram Ideogram Communication (Pic) symbols drawn in white on a black background; used in teaching Augmentative Communication, Gestural-Assisted (aided).

Picsyms. A set of symbols containing line drawings that can be used to teach nonoral expression of nouns, verbs, prepositions, and so forth; each symbol also is associated with printed English word; an open-ended system to which the clinician can add her own drawings; used in teaching Augmentative Communication, Gestural-Assisted (aided).

Pictographic Symbols. Pictorial representation of objects and events; easier to learn than abstract symbols; used in teaching Augmentative Communication, Gestural-Assisted (aided).

Pneumatic Device for Alaryngeal Speech. Sound source for patients with laryngectomy that uses the patient's exhaled air; a nonelectronic device one end of which is placed in the mouth and the other end is placed over the stoma; a vibrating reed in between provides sound that the patient articulates into speech; contrasted with Electronic Devices for Alaryngeal Speech.

Polyps. Protruding, soft, fluid-filled growths on the inner margin of the vocal folds; result of vocal abuse, often from a single abusive episode; often unilateral; may be *sessile* (broad-based) or *pedunculated* (the mass of the polyp connected to the vocal fold by a stalk-like structure); associated with hoarseness and breathiness; surgically removed.

- Identify the vocally abusive behaviors
- Reduce vocally abusive behaviors

Population. A large, defined group with certain characteristics identified for the purposes of a study; part of the Group Design Strategy of research; a representative Sample is randomly drawn from the population.

- Identify a large group of persons with defined characteristics (persons who stutter, people who have aphasia with additional defined characteristics relative to age, gender, severity, etc.)
- Randomly draw a sample of subjects needed for the study

Positive Practice. Required and unreinforced practice of a desirable behavior following Restitution for an undesirable behavior; one of the Direct Methods of Response Reduction; a part of Imposition of Work.

Positive Reinforcers. Events that, when presented immediately after a response is made, increase the future probability of that response; used extensively in communication training.

- Present potential reinforcer immediately after the correct response is made
- Use a Continuous Reinforcement schedule in the beginning and an Intermittent Reinforcement schedule subsequently

Prefer Conditioned Generalized Reinforcers, (e.g., Tokens) to Primary Reinforcers

Always use verbal praise (even when you use other kinds)

Use a different event when the one selected does not increase the response rate

- Call an event a reinforcer only when it increases a response rate

Postreinforcement Pause. A period of no responding after receiving a reinforcer; markedly evident in Fixed Interval Schedule of reinforcement.

Posttests. Measures of behaviors established after completing an experimental or routine teaching program; compared with Pretests; in a group design study, help rule-out the influence of extraneous variables.

Pragmatic Structures. Aspects of appropriate language use in naturalistic communicative contexts; targets of language intervention; include such skills as Conversational Repair; Eye Contact; Narrative Skills, Topic Initiation, Topic Maintenance; and Turn Taking (all described under Language Disorders in Children; Treatment of Language Disorders: Specific Techniques or Programs).

Prephonation Airflow. A target behavior for people who stutter and those who exhibit hard glottal attacks; includes a slight exhalation before initiating phonation; for procedures, see Stuttering Treatment, Treatment of Stuttering: Specific Techniques or Programs; Airflow Management; and Voice Disorders; Treatment of Voice Disorders; Specific Normal Voice Facilitating Techniques; Whisper-Phonation Method.

Premack-type Symbols. Plastic shapes or tokens designed by David Premack to teach communication to chimpanzees; Noniconic symbols that may be used to teach communicative skills to nonspeech clients; used in teaching Augmentative Communication Gestural-Assisted (aided).

Pretests. Measures of behaviors established before starting an experimental or routine teaching program; compared with posttests; in a group design study, help rule out the influence of extraneous variables.

Primary Reinforcers. Reinforcers whose effects do not depend on past learning; often fulfill biological needs; contrasted with Conditioned, Secondary, or Social Reinforcers; also known as unconditioned reinforcers.

- Use primary reinforcers with infants, toddlers, and other children who do not respond well to Social Reinforcers
- Use with children who are mentally retarded and those who are minimally verbal
- Always combine with social reinforcers
- Gradually withdraw primary reinforcers and keep the clients on social reinforcers

Principles (of Treatment). Empirical rules from which treatment procedures are derived.

Probes. Procedures used to assess generalized production of clinically established responses; administered every time a few exemplars are trained to assess generalized productions; may be Intermixed Probes, Pure Probes, or Conversational Probes.

Probe Criterion. A rule that specifies when to terminate training at a given topographic level of training or on a specified target behavior.

- A 90% correct Intermixed Probe response rate at each topographic level of training may suggest that the training may be moved to the next level (e.g., from the word to the phrase level)
- A 90% correct Pure Probe response rate for a behavior at the conversational level may suggest that the behavior is sufficiently trained and that the training may move on to another target behavior.

Probe Recording Sheet. A prepared sheet for recording probe response rates.

- Design and use a probe recording sheet similar to the following; modify as found necessary

Name of the Client	Treatment Target
Clinician	Date
Probe Recording Sheet	
Stimulus Items	Responses: + (Correct), – (Incorrect), 0 (No response)
1.	
2.	
3.	
4.	

Procedures (of treatment). Technical operations the clinician performs to effect changes in the client behaviors; actions of clinicians; contrasted with Treatment Targets; in describing treatment procedures:

- Specify what you ought to do to achieve the treatment target
- Specify the target communication skills
- Describe the stimulus conditions you need to arrange
- Specify the kinds of feedback you should give to the client under the differing conditions of correct, incorrect, and lack of responses
- Clarify how you measure the skills during treatment to document progress
- Describe how you plan to promote generalized productions and maintenance over time and across situations
- Specify the follow-up and booster treatment procedures

Production Training. Treatment designed to teach a client to produce a specified speech or oral language target; contrasted with Perceptual Training or Auditory Discrimination Training; emphasis is on what the client ought to say rather than just listen or respond nonverbally.

- Model the target skills and ask the client to imitate your productions
- Evoke the target skills and ask the client to produce them

Program (of treatment). An overall description of target behaviors, treatment variables, measurement procedures, generalization measures, maintenance strategies, follow-up, and so forth.

Prolonged Speech. A stuttering treatment target; syllables are prolonged to reduce the rate of speech; for procedures see Stuttering, Treatment; Treatment of Stuttering: Specific Techniques or Programs.

Prompts. Special stimuli that increase the probability of a response; prompts may be verbal or nonverbal.

- Prompt promptly, as the client hesitates (e.g., in teaching naming in a client with aphasia: "What is this?" "The word starts with a /t/")
- Prompt more frequently in the beginning to reduce errors
- Prefer a subtle or short prompt to ones that are loud or long (e.g., in teaching a person who stutters to speak slowly: "Slower" instead of "Speak at a slower rate")
- Prefer a gesture to a verbal prompt (e.g., in teaching a person who stutters to speak slowly: make a hand gesture to suggest a slower rate)
- Use Partial Modeling as a prompt
- Fade prompts as the responses become more consistent

Pseudo Supraglottic Swallow. A procedure to protect the airway during swallowing; used with patients who have dysphagia.

- Ask the patient to inhale, and hold the breath
- Swallow
- Cough.

Pull-out Therapy Model. A special education service delivery model in which children are taken out of the classroom for special services, including speech-language services.

Punishment. Procedures of reducing undesirable behaviors by response-contingent presentation or withdrawal of stimuli; includes Direct Methods of Response Reduction and Indirect Methods of Response Reduction.

- Minimize the use of response reduction procedures
- Simplify the target response and shape it to avoid or reduce the use of punishers
- Let the positive/corrective ratio be in favor of the positive (more reinforcers than punishers)
- Prefer the indirect methods of response reduction in which you replace undesirable behaviors with desirable behaviors that you positively reinforce
- When the client's correct responses do not increase, change your treatment procedures
- Watch for potential undesirable Side-Effects of Punishment

Pure Probes. Procedures to assess generalized production with only untrained stimulus items; to be administered when the client has met the intermixed probe criterion, preferably toward the end of treatment.

- Prepare a Probe Recording Sheet on which you have at least 10 untrained exemplars (untrained words, phrases, or sentences that contain the target sound or language feature)
- Present each exemplar on discrete trials
- Provide no reinforcement or corrective feedback
- Calculate the percent correct probe responses rate
- Give additional training when an adopted probe criterion is not met (e.g., 90% accuracy)
- Move on to next level of training or to new target behaviors when the criterion is met

Pushing Approach. A voice therapy procedure to promote better vocal fold approximations in clients who have weakened or paralyzed folds; for procedures, see Voice Disorders, Specific Normal Voice Facilitating Techniques.

Random Assignment. A method of assigning subjects selected for a study to either the experimental or the control group without the experimenter bias; used in treatment research; part of the Group Design Strategy.

- Select subjects randomly
- Assign a number to each subject
- Assign every even-numbered subject to one group and every odd-numbered subject to the other group

Random Selection. A method of selecting subjects (clients) to evaluate treatment effects or efficacy; each potential subject has an equal chance of being selected for the study, hence no experimenter bias in subject selection; need a large number of potential subjects for the method to work; part of the Group Design Strategy.

- Identify a large number of potential subjects
- Assign a number to each subject
- Select the required number of subjects randomly (e.g., every second, every fourth, or every tenth person)

Rate Reduction. A rate of speech slower than the normal or below a client-specific baserate; a target in the treatment of several communicative disorders including Stuttering, Cluttering, and Dysarthria.

Ratio Strain. Reduction in response rate due to a sudden thinning of reinforcement.

- to avoid ratio strain, gradually increase the ratio of reinforcement

Rationalism. A philosophical position that reason and intellect is the source of knowledge, not sensory experience; contrasted with Empiricism; closely related to Nativism.

Rebuses. Pictures of objects and persons used in teaching Augmentative Communication Gestural-Assisted (aided); different from just pictures in that words and grammatic morphemes are combined with rebuses; Iconic easier than Noniconic symbol systems to learn.

Recast. A child language intervention procedure in which the clinician expands a child's utterance type into a different type of sentence; procedure described under Language Disorders in Children; Treatment of language Disorders: Specific Techniques or Programs.

Recombinative Generalization. A form of generalization of taught behaviors in which various combinations of new stimuli evoke differential responding; varied and novel sentences formed out of previously taught words exemplify recombinative generalization.

Recurrent Laryngeal Nerve Resection. A medical treatment procedure for adductor spasmodic dysphonia; the recurrent laryngeal nerve is unilaterally resectioned to paralyze one of the folds to prevent hyperadduction.

Reduced Modeling. The same as Partial Modeling.

Regulated Breathing. A stuttering treatment target; includes inhalation, a slight exhalation before initiating phonation, and reduced rate of speech; for procedures see Stuttering, Treatment; Treatment of Stuttering: Specific Techniques or Programs.

Reinforce. Strengthen, increase.

Reinforcement. A method of selecting and strengthening behaviors of individuals by arranging consequences under specific stimulus conditions; widely used in the treatment of communicative disorders.

Reinforcement Priming. Seeking reinforcers for one's own behaviors; useful strategy for the client to learn in getting parents, teachers, peers, and others to notice the production of clinically established behaviors in natural settings and thus get reinforced; part of Maintenance Strategy.

- Teach others to reinforce the client for the production of target behaviors established in the clinic

- Teach the client to draw attention to his or her desirable communicative behaviors from others
- Verify that others are indeed reinforcing the client when attention is drawn to the production of target behaviors (e.g., have the client or the family members maintain and present records of reinforcement delivery)

Reinforcement Withdrawal. Taking away reinforcers to decrease a response; one of the Direct Methods of Response Reduction; includes Response Cost and Time-Out.

Reinforcers. Events that follow behaviors and thereby increase the future probability of those behaviors; widely used in treating communicative disorders.

Select either the Primary, Secondary, Conditioned Generalized, Informative Feedback, or High Probability Behaviors to reinforce clinical targets

- Reinforce initially on a Continuous Reinforcement schedule
- Switch to an Intermittent Reinforcement schedule later
- Always use verbal (conditioned) reinforcers in conjunction with other types
- Teach the client's significant others to reinforce the skills you establish

Reliability. Consistency with which the same event is repeatedly measured; important in clinical work and clinical research; includes inter- and intraobserver reliability.

Interobserver Reliability. The extent to which two (or more) observers agree in measuring an event.

- Measure a behavior of interest with its location identified for a unit-by-unit analysis (count not only the behaviors being measured, but also their locations in transcribed speech samples)
- Have another trained observer measure in the same manner (unit-by-unit analysis)
- Score the total number of locations for which both of you agreed for an Agreement count (A)

- Count the total number of locations for which only one of you, not both of you scored the behavior (stuttering, pitch breaks, articulatory error) for a Disagreement count (D)
- Calculate the unit-by-unit Agreement Index by using the following formula: A/(A+D) × 100

Intraobserver Reliability. The extent to which the same observer repeatedly measures the same event consistently.

- Measure the behavior of interest using the unit-by-unit method
- Measure again by the same method
- Calculate the Agreement Index using the same formula as given under interobserver reliability.

Replication. Conducting repeated research to show that a given procedure works with different clients, in different settings, and for different clinicians; important in treatment efficacy research; includes direct replication and systematic replication; both designed to show treatment Generality; one of the Treatment Selection Criteria.

Direct Replication. The same investigator repeats the same treatment experiment in the same setting but with different subjects who have the same characteristics as the original subjects.

- Initially, show that a treatment works with some clients
- Select different clients who share the same personal (age, gender) and clinical characteristics (severity, age of onset) as the original subjects
- Repeat the treatment experiment
- Analyze the results to evaluate generality of the treatment method

Systematic Replication. The same or different investigators repeat a treatment experiment in different settings, with clients who have different characteristics than the original clients; may even include clients with totally different diagnoses.

- Initially, an investigator shows that a treatment is effective with a sample of clients

- The same or a different investigator repeats the treatment research with another sample, with different personal (gender, age, health) and clinical (severity, age of onset) characteristics, and in a different setting than the original
- The investigator analyzes the results to evaluate the broader generality of the treatment method

Response Class. A group of responses created by the same or similar contingencies; functionally, but not necessarily structurally, similar responses; good treatment targets because there is generalized production within a class and discrimination between classes.

Response Complexity. Different topographic levels of a target behavior; structural complexity of communicative behaviors typically create a sequence of treatment.

- Teach words before phrases
- Phrases before sentences
- Sentences before conversational speech

Response Cost. A direct response reduction strategy in which the production of each response scheduled for reduction results in the loss of a reinforcer. In the **Earn and Lose** variety, clients earn a token for every correct response and lose one for every incorrect response. In the **Lose-Only** variety, the client who receives unearned tokens at the beginning of a session loses one for every incorrect response.

Earn and Lose

- Give a token, to be exchanged for back-up reinforcers, for correct responses
- Take a token away each time the client produces an incorrect response
- Exchange the tokens the client still possesses for back-up reinforcers at the end of the session

Lose-Only

- Give a certain number of tokens at the beginning of a session

- Take a token away each time the client produces an incorrect response
- Exchange the tokens the client still possesses for back-up reinforcers at the end of the session

Response Generalization. Production of unreinforced (new, untrained) responses that are similar to trained responses; a goal of treatment; typically achieved through various strategies designed to promote Generalization because stimulus generalization in language training also involves response generalization.

Response Mode Generalization. Production of unreinforced responses in a mode not involved in training.

- Train skills in a certain mode (e.g., fluency in oral reading)
- Probe to assess generalized production (fluency in conversational speech)
- If there is no generalization, train the skills in that mode (fluency in conversational speech)

Response Recording Sheet. A prepared sheet for recording correct, incorrect, and no responses given in treatment sessions.

- Design and use a response recording sheet similar to the following; modify as necessary

Name of the Client	Treatment Target
Clinician	Date
Response Recording Sheet	
Stimulus Items	Responses: + (Correct), – (Incorrect), 0 (No response)
1.	
2.	
3.	
4.	

A collection of procedures that help decrease undesirable responses; include Direct Methods of Response Reduction and Indirect Methods of Response Reduction.

Response Substitution. Increase in an undesirable behavior when another behavior is reduced; exemplified by increased frequency of wiggling in the chair when a child's disruptive hand movements are reduced by a response reduction method.

- Apply a response reduction strategy to the newly emerged undesirable behavior
- Apply such strategies sequentially if you have to

Response Unit. A training target in the Paired Stimuli Approach to treating articulation disorders (described under Articulation and Phonological Disorders; Treatment of Articulation and Phonological Disorders: Specific Techniques or Programs); the client is asked to produce a key word and a target word as a single response unit (e.g., this-bus); the client earns one reinforcer only by correctly producing the target sound in both the words.

Restitution. An element of overcorrection in which the person eliminates the effects of his or her misbehavior and then improves the situation; described under Imposition of Work.

- Ask the child who disorganizes your stimulus materials to reorganize them
- Next, ask the child to organize the toys on the floor (the disorganized toys were not the child's making)

Reversed Imitation. Clinician's imitation of a child's utterance during indirect language stimulation; in the operant Imitation, it is the client who imitates and the clinician who models.

Right Hemisphere Syndrome. A syndrome of brain injury and its consequences sustained in the right cerebral hemisphere; may be caused by cerebrovascular accidents, tumors, head trauma, or various neurological diseases; associated with perceptual, attentional, emotional, and communicative deficits; varying degrees of functional involvement depending on the site, nature, and extent of damage.

Treatment: General Considerations

- Counsel the family about communication treatment soon after the onset
- Begin treatment as soon as it is practical
- Select the client-specific treatment targets that:
  - will result in the most improvement in family, social, and vocational communication
  - help build other, more advanced communication skills
  - help focus on communicative treatment targets (e.g., attentional deficits may have to be treated before other language skills) the clients can imitate
- Develop stimulus materials that:
  - range from simple to progressively more complex and from fewer to greater number of elements
  - are clear, unambiguous, and relatively concrete
  - are familiar, meaningful to the client, and attractive
- Establish baselines of target behaviors
- Provide extensive and intensive practice
- Be aware that there is no controlled clinical evidence to support the use of computerized cognitive rehabilitation programs
- Structure treatment sessions initially and loosen them as the client becomes more proficient in producing the target responses
- Use instructions, modeling, and prompts in all stages of treatment
- Fade the special antecedents used in early stages of treatment
- Shape the target behaviors
- Give prompt and effective feedback
- Work with the family members to promote generalization and maintenance

Treatment: Targets and Procedures

Treat Lack of Awareness of Problems Experienced

- Give immediate verbal feedback on errors
- Give visual feedback on errors
- Tape record and replay the speech to the client and discuss the errors
- Teach the client Self-Control (Self-Monitoring) skills

Treat Impaired Attention

- Shape sustained attending behaviors with changing criterion (Changing Criterion, Treatment Procedure)
- Reinforce the client for paying attention to the stimulus material and for maintaining eye contact
- Structure the initial treatment sessions and reduce distractions, including noise
- Give alerting stimuli before presenting the treatment stimuli (e.g., "Look at me" before modeling a response, "Get ready, here comes the next picture" before presenting the stimulus picture; touching the client before presenting a treatment stimulus)
- Draw attention before you speak to the client (e.g., "Listen, I am going to tell you something")
- Vary the treatment stimuli, drop unattractive stimuli, use clear and forceful stimuli
- Give frequent, brief breaks in the initial phase of treatment; reduce the number and duration of the breaks gradually
- Introduce gradually some distracting stimuli while still reinforcing attention to treatment tasks

Treat Visual Neglect

- Use printed material or any means that would force attention to the neglected side
- Teach the patient to keep a finger on the left margin while reading and track back to it before beginning a new line
- Color the left-side margins, draw a colored line through the margin, or use other discriminative stimuli to force attention to the left side of reading texts; fade such stimuli

- Tell the patient to "Look to the left" when the client reaches the end of sentences; fade such verbal cues
- Teach the clients to recognize what they read does not make sense; teach them to quiz themselves about what they read
- Design reading materials with large print and progressively smaller print and ask the client to read them aloud

Treat Impulsive Behaviors

- Teach the client to wait and withhold responses
- Give nonverbal signals to delay responses
- Fade the noverbal signals and introduce verbal signals to wait, withhold, and delay

Treat Pragmatic Language Skills

- Teach the client to initiate conversation; have the client discuss various topics in which you teach various skills by modeling them, ask the client to use them, and reinforce the client for using them; for instance:
  - teach the client to introduce the topic explicitly
  - teach the client to give background information on narratives and stories
  - teach the client to periodically restate the topic of discussion
  - prompt the client to maintain focus on the main topic
  - teach the client to ask such questions as "Do you follow me?" or "Do you understand?"
  - give corrective feedback
- Teach the client to request clarification when messages are not understood (e.g., "Please repeat that," or "I do not understand")
- Teach the client to maintain eye contact during conversation; use such verbal stimuli as "Look at me"
- Reinforce progressively longer durations of topic maintenance
- Teach the client to take turns in conversation; stop the client for inappropriate turn taking (e.g., interrupting you)

- Use the PACE program (Promoting Aphasics' Communicative Effectiveness; described under Aphasia; Treatment of Aphasia: Specific Techniques or Programs) for teaching social communication

Treat Impaired Reasoning Skills

- Teach the client to think and plan (e.g., discuss how the client might plan a vacation; help the client move in a logical manner)
- Pose different kinds of problems one might encounter in real life and ask the client to solve them (e.g., "How do you buy an airplane ticket?")

Treat Impaired Inference

- Tell stories and ask questions to evoke implied information
- Describe situations that require the client to draw logical conclusions

Treat Impaired Recognition of Absurdities

- Show pictures that depict logical and absurd events and ask the client to separate them (e.g., picture of a cat chasing a rat and picture of a rat chasing a cat)
- Present verbal or written statements that are logical or absurd and ask the client to separate them
- Ask the client to explain why a statement is absurd or logical

Treat Impaired Comprehension of Metaphors or Idioms

- Ask the client to select statements that give literal meanings
- Asking the client to sort out literal and figurative statements
- Set up hypothetical situations that require such judgments

Treat Comprehension of Figurative Meanings

- Begin with nonliteral meanings that the client presently uses and understands
- Provide multiple meanings for a single statement

- Discuss the difference between what the statement apparently says and what it means
- Use stimuli that the client was familiar with and used premorbidly

Treat Comprehension of Humor

- Associate captions with cartoons
- Link the punchline with the body of the joke

Teach Compensatory Strategies

- Monitor the comprehension of the speaker's utterance
- Teach the use of such functional memory aids as lists of things do, writing down appointments, having a checklist of things to do before leaving the house, keeping related things together, and so forth
- Teach Self-Control (Self-Monitoring) skills including the generation of memory aids
- Teach the client to stop and self-correct when errors are made
- Make a few socially appropriate and inappropriate statements and ask the client to evaluate them
- Have the client evaluate social appropriateness of his or her own productions
- Teach the client to rephrase inappropriate comments to make them more appropriate

Brookshire, R. H. (1992). *An introduction to neurogenic communication disorders* (4th ed.). St. Louis, MO: Mosby Year Book.

Hegde, M. N. (1994). *A coursebook on aphasia and other neurogenic language disorders*. San Diego, CA: Singular Publishing Group.

Tompkins, C. A. (1995). *Right hemisphere communication disorders: Theory and management*. San Diego, CA: Singular Publishing Group.

Rigidity. Stiffness of muscles and joints.

Sample. A smaller number of individuals selected from a larger population for a research study.

Satiation. Temporary termination of a drive or need because it has been satisfied; a potential problem with Primary Reinforcers (e.g., food).

- Give only small amounts of food or drink to reinforce individual responses
- Let the client accumulate food that he or she can eat later
- Arrange treatment sessions, especially with infants and toddlers who need primary reinforcers, around breakfast or lunch time
- Ask parents to withhold the primary reinforcers you plan to use before coming to treatment sessions

Scanning in Augmentative Communication. message-election method in augmentative communication; the clinician or a conversational partner offers various choices available on a message display (e.g., a communication board) until the client signals the right choice; the communication partner, for example, may point to different messages until the client indicates that a particular message pointed to is the one intended.

Schedules of Reinforcement. Different patterns of reinforcement that generate different patterns of responses; include Continuous Reinforcement schedules and Intermittent Reinforcement schedules.

- Use continuous reinforcement schedule in the beginning of treatment
- Shift to an intermittent schedule as learning becomes more stable

Science. A certain philosophy of nature and events which includes Determinism and Empiricism, a particular disposition exhibited by scientists (e.g., valuing evidence more than opinions), and a set of methods used in investigating events (objective, experimental).

Script. A presumed mental representation of repeatedly occurring, sequenced events, episodes, or personal experiences; used in teaching advanced language skills including narrative skills; a description of baking cookies or running a hot dog stand is a script; it has a beginning and an end, actions people take, or roles people play; for procedures, see Language Disorders in Children; Treatment of Language Disorders: Specific Techniques or Programs.

Script Therapy. The use of Scripts in teaching language skills to children with language impairment; for procedures, see Language Disorders in Children; Treatment of Language Disorders: Specific Techniques or Programs.

Secondary Reinforcers. Conditioned reinforcers whose effects depend on past learning; appropriate reinforcers for all kinds of verbal responses except for certain kinds of mands that request food and drink; include Social Reinforcers, Conditioned Generalized Reinforcers, Informative Feedback, and High Probability Behaviors.

Self-Control. A behavior that monitors and modifies other behaviors of the same person; a necessary skill in maintaining clinically acquired communicative behaviors.

Self-Control (Self-Monitoring) Teaching Procedures. Techniques of monitoring one's own behavior to effect significant and positive changes; useful to teach these techniques to clients within a Maintenance Strategy.

- Teach clients to discriminate their own incorrect and undesirable responses
- Teach them to contrast their desirable and undesirable responses
- Teach them to measure their behaviors reliably
- Let clients measure their behaviors along with you in treatment sessions
- Give them frequent feedback on their measurement to improve their skill

- Teach clients to monitor their behaviors by measuring them outside the clinic
- Teach them to generate signals for their own actions (e.g., written notes, wristwatch reminders, asking others to help monitor their behaviors)
- Teach clients to pause after they produce a wrong response
- Teach clients to correct their own mistakes or nontarget responses
- Teach clients to anticipate problems and take corrective actions
- In group therapy, teach clients to correct other participants' errors

Self Talk. A child language intervention procedure in which the clinician describes his or her own activity while playing with a child; procedure described under Language Disorders in Children; Treatment of Language Disorders: Specific Techniques or Programs.

Sequence of Treatment. Movement within a treatment program from the beginning to the end; a description of steps involved in implementing a treatment plan; progression of treatment from a simple to a more complex level; see Treatment in Communicative Disorders, General Sequence.

Service Delivery Models. Different arrangements of providing assessment and treatment services to children with communication disorders, include the Collaborative Model, the Consultant Model, the Language-Based Classroom Model, and the Pull-Out Therapy Model.

Shaping. A method of teaching nonexistent responses that are not even imitated; also known as successive approximation.

- Select a target response (the terminal response)
- Simplify that target behavior
- Identify an initial response the client can imitate
- Identify intermediate responses
- Teach the initial response; in successive stages, teach the intermediate responses

- Continue until the terminal response is taught

Side-Effects of Punishment. Undesirable effects of punishment procedures; include emotional reactions, aggressive reactions, unexpected increase in the punished response, increase in a different response than the one punished, and so forth; to be eliminated or minimized by prudent use of response reduction methods.
- Always use positive reinforcers for desirable behaviors
- Keep reinforcement:punishment ratio in favor of reinforcement
- Shape a difficult response to avoid using response reduction methods
- Consistently apply response reduction methods to all undesirable behaviors
- Remove or reduce reinforcement for undesirable behaviors
- Never associate response reduction methods with positive reinforcement

Sig Symbols. A set of pictographic or ideographic symbols based on American Sign Language; used on communication boards; used in teaching Augmentative Communication Gestural-Assisted (aided).

Significant Others. People who typically interact with a client on a daily basis; include family members, teachers, friends, colleagues, baby sitters, and healthcare workers; important in helping the client learn and maintain communicative behaviors; recipients of training within a Maintenance Strategy.

Single-Subject Design Strategy. Methods of demonstrating treatment effects by showing contrasts between conditions of no treatment, treatment, withdrawal of treatment, and other control procedures; typically, all subjects selected receive treatment (no control group); includes, among others, ABA Design, ABAB Design, and Multiple Baseline Design; contrasted with Group Design Strategy.

Social Reinforcers. A variety of conditioned reinforcers frequently used in treatment sessions; include verbal praise, attention, touch, eye contact, and facial expressions; resistant to satiation effect; may not work with nonverbal clients.

- With children who are nonverbal, profoundly retarded, and very young (infants and toddlers), pair social reinforcers with primary reinforcers
- Eventually, fade the primary reinforcers and maintain the responses on social reinforcers only

Soft Articulatory Contacts. A stuttering treatment target; includes relaxed, easy, and soft contact of articulators in speech production; used in conjunction with such other techniques as Airflow Management and Rate Reduction; for procedures see Stuttering, Treatment; Treatment of Stuttering: Specific Techniques or Programs.

Spasmodic Dysphonia. A voice disorder characterized in most cases by severe overadduction of vocal folds and strained or choked-off voice quality; phonation may be impossible; in other cases, characterized by sudden abduction of folds and resulting aphonia; of unknown etiology; possible neuropathology; voice therapy is not particularly helpful.

Spastic Dysarthria. A type of motor speech disorder; its neuropathology is bilateral damage to the upper motor neuron (direct and indirect motor pathways) resulting in weakness, spastic paralysis, limited range of movement, and slowness of movement; may affect all aspects of speech and usually not confined to one aspect; major speech problems include strained-strangled-harsh voice, hypernasality, slow rate, consonant imprecision, and monopitch and monoloudness; select appropriate treatment targets and procedures described under Dysarthria, Treatment; in addition, consider the following that apply especially to spastic dysarthria:

- Consult with the client's physician about medically controlling pathological crying which might interfere with treatment

- Consider behaviorally modifying crying in treatment sessions by reinforcing noncrying (alternative) behaviors
- Do not teach pushing or pulling exercises that only aggravate hyperadduction
- Use relaxation and stretching exercises with caution because their effects on speech have not been documented

Duffy, J. R. (1995). *Motor speech disorders.* St. Louis, MO: C.V. Mosby.

Johns, D. F. (Ed.). (1985). *Clinical management of neurogenic communicative disorders.* Boston: Little, Brown.

Yorkston, K. M., Beukelman, D. R., & Bell, K. R. (1988). *Clinical management of dysarthric speakers.* Austin, TX: Pro-Ed.

Specific Language Impairment (SLI). Language disorders in children who are otherwise normal, although some may have subtle cognitive deficits; different language skills may be somewhat differentially affected; pragmatic skills may be better than syntactic and morphological skills; a diagnosis made on negative grounds (no other factor, such as mental retardation or neurologic deficits, explains the disorder); some believe that SLI suggests limited language skills with no pathology; treatment procedures the same as those for Language Disorders in Children.

Specific Normal Voice Facilitating Techniques. A collection of voice therapy procedures used to promote normal voice productions; see Voice Disorders; Specific Normal Voice Facilitating Techniques.

Stimulus Generalization. Production of a newly learned response to stimuli not used in training; an important goal of intervention.

- Use a variety of stimuli during treatment
- Use common stimuli
- Ask clients to bring objects, toys, books and so forth from home to use as stimuli

Stimulation Versus Treatment or Teaching. In language intervention, stimulation tends to be less directed, more naturalistic, without specific language targets, without a requirement that the child imitate modeled responses, and is often implemented by nonclinicians; treatment or teaching tends to be more clinician-directed, less naturalistic, with specific language structures as targets, with the requirement that the child imitate modeled responses, and often implemented by speech-language pathologists.

Stimulus Withdrawal. A group of procedures used to reduce incorrect responses during treatment; a reinforcer or a reinforcing state of affairs is removed as soon as an incorrect response is made; includes Time-Out and Response-Cost.

Story Grammar. The structure of narratives which may be treatment targets for children with language disorders; described under Language Disorders in Children; Treatment of Language Disorders: Specific Techniques or Programs.

Stridency. A voice disorder characterized by an unpleasant, shrill, and metallic-sounding voice; caused by excessive pharyngeal constriction and an elevated larynx.

- Use the Chewing Method
- Model and contrast good vocal production with a strident production
- Lower the pitch; use Glottal Fry
- Teach relaxation
- Teach oral openness
- Use Yawn-Sigh method

Stuttering. A disorder of fluency characterized by excessive amounts of Dysfluencies, excessive durations of dysfluencies, and unusual amount of muscular effort in speaking; has varied definitions including an involuntary loss of speech motor control, part-word repetitions and sound prolongations, efforts to avoid stuttering, a social role conflict, and so forth; may be associated with avoidance of certain words and speaking situations; experience of negative emotions and expression of negative verbalizations about him- or herself and about listeners.

Stuttering, Treatment. Stuttering has varied treatment procedures; only a few have been tested for their efficacy; some are questionable; some have uncontrolled clinical support; several are purely rational; most clinicians combine certain effective components of treatment to create somewhat personal programs; airflow management, gentle phonatory onset, and rate reduction through prolonged syllables are common elements across diverse contemporary treatment programs; these programs are empirically supported with some experimental evidence.

1. A contemporary, integrated, comprehensive treatment procedure for stuttering in older children and adults

- Make a thorough assessment; determine the forms and the frequencies of stuttering in both conversational speech and oral reading in clinical and extraclinical situations
- Baserate stuttering in the clinic
- Select the three target fluency skills that are incompatible with stuttering, commonly used, and known to be effective in establishing stutter-free speech: Airflow Management, Gentle Phonatory Onset, and Rate Reduction through syllable prolongation; all described later under Treatment of Stuttering: Specific Techniques or Programs.
- Counsel the client and the family about the treatment program, its known effects, its drawback (initially unacceptable, artificial fluency), and the potential need for Booster Therapy in the future
- Initially, teach one target skill at a time; complete this component training in one session
- Model airflow management
  - inhale a slightly deeper than usual amount of air through your nose
  - exhale a slight amount of air through your open mouth
- Ask the client to imitate your airflow modeling
- Reinforce correct imitated responses promptly
- Stop the client at the earliest sign of mismanaged airflow; pause briefly and continue

- Continue until the client can, upon request and without modeling, inhale through the nose and exhale a slight amount of air through the mouth
- Model gentle phonatory onset; add it to the airflow component
  - initiate syllables softly, gently, slowly, and in a relaxed manner only after the inhalation and slight exhalation
- Ask the client to imitate your modeling of airflow management and gentle phonatory onset
- Reinforce correct imitations promptly
- Stop the client at the earliest sign of mismanaged airflow, abrupt or tensed onset of phonation, or stuttering (dysfluency); pause briefly and continue
- Continue until the client can, upon request and without modeling, inhale, exhale a slight amount, and initiate syllables softly and gently
- Model rate reduction through syllable prolongation; add it to airflow management and gentle phonatory onset; prefer the clinician-induced rate reduction; use Delayed Auditory Feedback if necessary (described later under Treatment of Stuttering: Specific Techniques or Programs).
  - begin at the word level
  - model stretched-out syllable durations with continuous phonation
- Ask the client to imitate your modeling of all three target skills
- Reinforce correct imitations of airflow management, gentle phonatory onset, and syllable prolongations
- Use oral reading initially to stabilize the production of all three target behaviors
- Stop the client for mismanaged targets or production of stuttering; pause briefly and continue
- Continue until the client can produce all three target behaviors upon request and without modeling and with stutter-free speech at the word level with 98 to 100% accuracy
- Shift training to the phrase level

- integrate all three skills
- model as often as is necessary
- fade modeling
- promptly reinforce for correct productions of phrases with inhalation and slight exhalation, gentle phonatory onset, and rate reduction through syllable prolongation
- stop the client for mismanagement of any of the targets and production of dysfluencies; pause briefly and continue

- Shift training to the sentence level
  - model and have the client imitate sentences if necessary; target completely stutter-free productions
  - ask questions the client will answer with complete sentences; monitor all target behaviors and fluency
  - stop the client for mismanagement of any of the targets and production of dysfluencies
  - continue until the client speaks in sentences with stutter-free speech by using airflow management, gentle phonatory onset, and rare reduction through syllable prolongation
- Shape normal prosody
  - model a slightly higher speech rate and ask the client to imitate it
  - ask the client to speak at progressively higher rate while maintaining stutter-free speech
  - model pitch variations and let the client imitate and then talk spontaneously with increased intonational patterns
  - model appropriate vocal intensity and let the client imitate and then talk with sufficient loudness
  - make continuous judgments about speech naturalness and modify the speech to approximate normal prosodic features
  - reinforce all appropriate productions
  - stop the client for excessively slow rate and monotonous speech; pause and continue
  - continue until the speech is judged both normally fluent and natural-sounding
- Implement a maintenance program

- teach the client Self-Control (Self-Monitoring) skills by having him or her count dysfluencies, the production of target behaviors, increase in rate, abrupt phonatory onset, and breath holding
- teach the client to stop talking and to pause briefly when he or she stutters or mismanages a target skill
- hold informal treatment sessions in naturalistic settings
- signal the client in a subtle manner to use the target skills
- train the family members, teachers, friends, colleagues, and others in prompting and reinforcing the production of target skills and fluency
- train teachers and family members to provide opportunities to practice fluency skills
- train family members to hold informal treatment sessions at home

- Dismiss the client only when natural sounding fluency is established in natural settings and in conversational speech
- Counsel the client and the family about the potential for relapse and the need for booster treatment
- Follow-up and arrange for booster treatment

2. *A contemporary, integrated, comprehensive treatment procedure for stuttering in very young children (2 to 5 year olds)*

- Make a thorough assessment; determine the forms and the frequencies of stuttering in both conversational speech and oral reading in clinical and extraclinical situations
- Baserate stuttering in the clinic
- Use toys, objects, pictures, storybooks, and a loosely structured play situation to evoke and manage speech from the child
- Experiment informally with all three targets used with older children and adults: airflow management, gentle phonatory onset, and rate reduction through syllable prolongation; possibly, with very young children only a slower rate may be effective in inducing stutter-free speech; if

so, skip the others; most likely to be skipped is airflow management; the next most likely to be skipped is gentle phonatory onset; the younger the child, the more likely it is that you will use only slow speech

- Counsel the family about the treatment program, its known effects, its drawback (initially unacceptable, artificial fluency), and the potential need for booster therapy in the future; impress on them the need to regularly work with the child at home and the critical role they play in fluency maintenance
- Even if you use gentle phonatory onset and airflow management, emphasize slow normal speech; if you use all three, teach one target skill at a time; refer to the preceding program for steps involved in implementing the optional airflow management and gentle phonatory onset; model more frequently and use simple language with younger children
- Model rate reduction through syllable prolongation; use a rubber band to show stretching of syllables; use hand gestures to slow speech; use any other means the child will comprehend; model more frequently than you would for older children and adults; reduce your own rate; if selected, add rate reduction to airflow management and gentle phonatory onset; do not use DAF with very young children
  - begin at the word level
  - model stretched-out syllable durations with continuous phonation
- Ask the child to imitate your modeling
- Reinforce correct imitations
- Stop the child for mismanaged targets or production of stuttering; pause briefly and continue
- Continue until the child can produce slow speech (or with the optional targets) upon request and without modeling and with stutter-free speech at the word level with 98 to 100% accuracy

- Shift training to the phrase level
  - model often
  - fade modeling
  - promptly reinforce stutter-free production of phrases
  - stop the child for mismanagement of the target or targets and production of dysfluencies; pause briefly and continue
- Shift training to the sentence level
  - model frequently and have the child imitate sentences; target completely stutter-free productions
  - ask questions the child will answer with complete sentences; monitor target behavior or behaviors and fluency
  - stop the child for mismanagement of the target or targets and production of dysfluencies
  - continue until the child speaks in sentences with stutter-free speech
- Shape normal prosody
  - model a slightly higher speech rate and ask the child to imitate it
  - encourage the child to speak at progressively higher rate while maintaining stutter-free speech
  - model pitch variations and let the child imitate and then talk spontaneously with increased intonational patterns
  - model appropriate vocal intensity and let the child imitate and then talk with sufficient loudness
  - make continuous judgments about speech naturalness and modify the speech to approximate normal prosodic features
  - reinforce all appropriate productions
  - stop the child for excessively slow rate and monotonous speech; pause and continue
  - continue until the speech is judged both normally fluent and natural-sounding
- Implement a maintenance program
  - teach the client to stop talking and to pause briefly when he or she stutters or mismanages the target skill or skills

- hold informal treatment sessions in naturalistic settings
- signal the client in a subtle manner to use the target skills
- train the family members, babysitters, preschool teachers, and day care workers in prompting and reinforcing slow, normal, and fluent speech in the child
- train teachers and family members to provide opportunities to practice fluency skills
- ask parents to participate in all treatment sessions you conduct
- train family members to evoke a slow, normal rate of speech and to positively reinforce fluency
- ask them to withhold random, noncontingent negative feedback to the child
- teach them the skills of gently stopping the child when stuttering occurs and to pause and continue
- teach parents to hold informal treatment sessions at home; ask them to submit tape recorded sessions for your analysis and feedback to the parents
- teach the parents to monitor fluency in a subtle and nonpunitive manner most of the time

- Dismiss the child only when natural sounding fluency is established in natural settings and in conversational speech
- Counsel the family about the potential for relapse and the need for booster treatment
- Follow-up and arrange for booster treatment

Treatment of Stuttering: Specific Techniques or Programs

Airflow Management in Stuttering Treatment. Regulated use of airflow used in the treatment of stuttering; also called Regulated Breathing; a component in many stuttering treatment procedures; effective in inducing stutter-free speech; supported by clinical research; often combined with other treatment targets including Gentle Phonatory Onset and Prolonged Speech (described later in this section).

- Preferably, combine it with prolonged speech and gentle phonatory onset

- Model Regulated Breathing to produce stutter-free speech
  - take an inhalation through the nose, slightly deeper than the usual so it is easily observed
  - exhale a small amount of air through the mouth before initiating phonation
  - initiate phonation slowly, gently, and softly only after the start of exhalation
  - model the production of single words or phrases
  - prolong the vowels and reduce the rate
- Ask the client to imitate your modeled productions
- Reinforce the imitative productions
- Model frequently and stabilize regulated breathing of inhalation and slight prevoice exhalation
- Fade modeling and evoke regulated breathing and speech production
- Move through the sequence of words, phrases, and sentences as you add other components (soft and gentle phonatory onset, prolongation of vowels, and slow rate of speech)
- Fade the explicit management of airflow into a more natural use of airflow to sustain fluency in conversational speech in and out of the clinic
- Reinstate regulated breathing throughout the treatment when found necessary

Continuous Airflow. Maintaining airflow throughout an utterance; in conjunction with such other treatment targets as rate reduction, helps induce stutter-free speech.

- Instruct the client to take enough air before beginning speech production
- Ask the client to exhale a slight amount of air before initiating phonation
- Ask the client to initiate phonation gently and softly
- Ask the client to maintain an even airflow throughout an utterance
- Model the technique

- Reinforce the client for correct production of the target behavior

Continuous Phonation. Maintaining phonation throughout an utterance; a stuttering treatment target; often combined with Gentle Phonatory Onset, Airflow Management, and Prolonged Speech (all described in this section).

- Instruct the client in maintaining phonation throughout an utterance
- Model continuous phonation in such a way as to blur the word boundaries
- Ask the client to imitate your modeling
- Reinforce correctly imitated productions
- Begin with shorter phrases and progress to longer sentences
- Combine it with other targets, including syllable prolongation, gentle phonatory onset, and airflow management

Counseling as Treatment for Stuttering. A collection of varied approaches to treating stuttering by giving information, advice, and strategies to deal with the problem; a range of techniques most of them psychologically oriented; recipients are parents of children who stutter and adults who stutter; often combined with direct methods of treating stuttering; efficacy of counseling when used exclusively with no direct work with stuttering by either the clinician or the parent is not established; when combined with direct work on stuttering, whether counseling had any effect is unclear.

Counseling Parents of Children Who Stutter. Using the psychological methods of counseling to indirectly treat stuttering in their children; an Indirect Stuttering Treatment method (described later in this section); the main approach is talking with the child's parents to change their feelings, attitudes, ideas, and expectations about stuttering and fluency; efficacy of this approach not established; often combined with Direct Stuttering Treatment (described later in this section).

- Be a sensitive, noncritical, accepting listener
- Find out what the parents wish to accomplish through counseling
- Let the parents explore their feelings, emotions, perceptions, and expectations relative to their child's stuttering
- Let the parents freely talk about their fears, possible feelings of guilt, and their overt reactions to stuttering in their child
- Let the parents talk about their strategies of dealing with stuttering in their child
- Help the parents find their own solutions by offering professional views and ideas they may not have known or considered
- Express approval of their positive feelings and helpful reactions toward their child
- Help them realize their child's strengths and limitations
- Reduce their negative thoughts and feelings, including potential feelings of guilt by reassuring them that they may not have created the problem
- Let the parents put their child's stuttering in a perspective so that they do not exaggerate its negative effects
- Let the parents realize that no child is fluent all the time
- Explore actions the parents may have taken with positive effects on the child's fluency and encourage them to increase or strengthen them
- Explore actions the parents may have taken that have worsened the child's problems and encourage them to eliminate or reduce them
- Explore the parents' ideas about fluency and stuttering to encourage a more realistic views of them

- Discuss the kinds of communicative demands the parents make and ask them to reduce such demands
- Encourage the parents to create more positive speech experiences for the child by withholding criticism and accepting the child's stuttered attempts at communication

Counseling Persons Who Stutter. Using psychological methods of counseling to indirectly treat persons who stutter; an Indirect Stuttering Treatment (described later in this section); the main approach is talking with the client to change feelings, attitudes, and expectations; efficacy of this approach not established; often combined with Direct Stuttering Treatment (described later in this section).

- Be a sensitive, noncritical, accepting listener
- Find out what the client wishes to accomplish through counseling
- Let the client explore his or her feelings, emotions, perceptions, and expectations relative to stuttering
- Let the client talk about the difficult speaking situations, listener reactions, and his or her own emotional reactions
- Help the client find his or her own solutions by offering professional views and ideas the client may be unaware or may not have considered
- Discuss the client's strengths that he or she may not have realized
- Reduce negative thoughts and feelings by having the client concentrate on positive experiences, including positive speech experiences
- Let the client put stuttering in a perspective so that he or she does not exaggerate its negative effects
- Let the client realize that no one is fluent all the time

- Explore actions the client takes that may exacerbate stuttering and encourage to eliminate or reduce them
- Explore actions and situations that enhance fluency and encourage to increase them or strengthen them
- Encourage the client to talk more positively about him- or herself

Delayed Auditory Feedback (DAF). Hearing one's own speech after a delay introduced by a mechanical device; most typical effect is to slow down the rate of speech; used in treating persons who stutter and those who clutter to slow their speech rate; reduces or eliminates stuttering, but induces unnatural sounding speech; a widely used stuttering treatment technique; a component in many programmed or comprehensive treatment approaches; useful in establishing Stutter-Free Speech (described later in this section) but needs additional procedures to make the speech sound natural and to make the fluency last over time and across situations.

- Assess the client thoroughly and establish baserates of stuttering and the speech rate
- Select a miniaturized, electronic feedback devise that the client can use in most situations
- Ask the client to wear the portable device (may use a desk-top unit with a loss in flexibility)
- Experiment with different delays to set a client-specific delay that induces stutter-free speech (most clients are stutter-free at 250 milliseconds of delay)
- Begin by asking the client to respond to questions that evoke two- or three-word phrases or short sentences
- Drop down to word level only if the client cannot maintain stutter-free speech at the phrase or short-sentence level
- Model slow, prolonged speech if necessary
- Use oral reading to stabilize a slow, prolonged production if necessary (some initially find oral reading under DAF easier than speaking)

- Establish stutter-free speech with the initial delay over a few sessions
- Increase the length of utterances gradually
- Move to more spontaneous conversational speech containing longer and more complex utterances
- Fade the DAF by decreasing the delay in gradual steps; reduce it in 50 millisecond intervals or other intervals that still help maintain stutter-free speech
- Reduce the intensity of DAF
- Increase the rate of speech while still maintaining stutter-free speech; reinforce the client for speaking at progressively faster rates
- Eliminate the delay altogether, but let the client wear the unit
- Increase the rate further to move it closer to the pre-treatment, judged normal, or natural sounding rate
- Shape the normal prosodic features including normal rhythm, intonation, intensity variations, emotional connotations, and so forth
- Conduct informal treatment sessions in varied non-clinical settings
- Train family members, teachers, and others to reinforce fluent, natural sounding speech in nonclinical settings
- Teach Self-Control (Self-Monitoring) skills (charting one's own stuttering, stopping soon after a stuttering or at the earliest sign of increased rate)
- Dismiss only after a natural sounding fluent speech is established
- Counsel the client about the possibility of relapse and the need for Booster Treatment
- Follow-up and arranger for booster treatment (relapses are common; follow-up and booster treatment are critical in maintenance)

Direct Stuttering Reduction Strategy: Response Cost. Withdrawal of a positive reinforcer made contingent on stuttering; each stuttering costs the client a reinforcer he or she has access to; effective in reducing stuttering; supported by controlled experimental evidence; especially applicable with children; does not induce an artificial pattern of fluency that should be faded out.

- Assess the client thoroughly and establish baserates of stuttering or dysfluencies, as defined
- Use pictures, objects, storybooks, and toys to evoke continuous speech from young children,
- Use topic cards initially to promote extended monologues from adults
- Introduce natural conversation with both adults and children as soon as practical
- Instruct the client about the procedure: " I will give you a token for every word *(later phrases and sentences)* you speak without stuttering. At the end of the session, you can exchange the tokens for this gift here. You should at least have five tokens *(or any such low number that ensures the gift for the child)* at the end of the session. The main thing is that I will take a token away from you every time you stutter. You should try to keep as many tokens as possible by speaking without stuttering."
- Ask the child to state the rule and repeat the instructions if necessary
- Reinforce initially for every fluently spoken word; progress to phrases, controlled sentences, and conversational speech
- Take a token away promptly and in a matter-of-fact manner immediately following a stuttering or at the earliest sign of it
- Watch for undue emotional responses at token loss; they tend to disappear; however, if they persist, switch to another procedure
- Measure the frequency of stutterings or dysfluencies as you have defined them in each session or after the session through tape-recorded samples

- Teach Self-Control (Self-Monitoring) skills in which the client measures and records his or her stutterings and learns to hand you a token at the earliest sign of stuttering (self-imposed response-cost)
- Fade response cost and keep the client on social, verbal reinforcers for fluency
- Train family members, teachers, siblings, friends, and others to give subtle signals for the client to stop when they observe stuttering in all situations
- Shift treatment to naturalistic settings; give unobtrusive feedback to the client in such settings
- Train parents or spouses to hold informal training sessions; let them initially use your token system; later let them fade the tokens and use only verbal praise
- Have the client or the family members submit tape-recorded home conversational speech samples for your analysis of stuttering frequency
- Dismiss the client only when the rate of dysfluencies is below the set criterion (e.g., less than 3%)
- Counsel the client, family members, or both about possible relapse of stuttering and the need for booster treatment; ask the client to contact you as soon as there is an increase in stuttering
- Follow-up the client and arrange for booster treatment

Direct Stuttering Reduction Strategy: Time-out. A brief period of nonreinforcement during which the client stops talking and the clinician avoids eye contact with the client; the period is imposed at the earliest sign of an imminent stuttering or associated behaviors or immediately following those behaviors; duration typically does not exceed 10 seconds; effective in reducing stuttering; supported by controlled experimental evidence; has the advantage of not inducing an artificial and unacceptable pattern of fluency; especially effective with children.

- Assess the client thoroughly and baserate stuttering or dysfluencies, as defined

- Use pictures, objects, storybooks, and toys to evoke continuous speech from young children,
- Use topic cards initially to promote extended monologues from adults
- Introduce natural conversation with both adults and children as soon as practical
- Instruct the client about the procedure: "I will be saying 'Stop' at the earliest sign of stuttering. I want you to stop talking immediately. I will also look away from you and count to 5 seconds. I will then look at you again. When I look at you, continue talking."
- Ask the child to state the rule and repeat the instructions if necessary
- At the earliest sign of stuttering, say "Stop," look away for 5 seconds, and then reestablish eye contact
- If the client does not begin talking immediately, prompt verbally or nonverbally (e.g., "You were telling me"; "Yes, continue"; a hand gesture to continue)
- Stop the client for every instance of stuttering or dysfluencies; be prompt, forceful, and unambiguous in your feedback
- Ensure that the client does stop talking when you say so
- Watch for undue emotional responses; they tend to disappear; however, if they persist, switch to another procedure
- Measure the frequency of stutterings or dysfluencies as you have defined them in each session or after the session through tape-recorded samples
- Begin with words and phrases and progress to controlled sentences and natural conversational speech
- Teach Self-Control (Self-Monitoring) skills in which the client measures and records his or her stutterings and learns to pause at the earliest sign of stuttering (self-imposed time-out)

- Train family members, teachers, siblings, friends, and others to give subtle signals for the client to stop when they observe stuttering in all situations
- Fade time-out and keep the client on social, verbal reinforcers for fluency
- Shift treatment to naturalistic settings; give unobtrusive feedback to the client in such settings
- Train parents or spouses to hold informal training sessions at home; let them use time-out initially for stuttering and only verbal praise for fluency later
- Have the client or the family members submit tape-recorded home conversational speech samples for your analysis of stuttering frequency
- Dismiss the client only when the rate of dysfluencies is below the set criterion (e.g., less than 3%)
- Counsel the client, the family members, or both about possible relapse of stuttering and the need for booster treatment; ask the client to contact you as soon as stuttering increases
- Follow-up the client and arrange for booster treatment

Direct Stuttering Treatment. Methods in which the clinician concentrates on reducing stuttering in the client as against trying to indirectly reduce it through counseling and other methods; in behavioral treatment, includes <u>Direct Stuttering Reduction Strategy: Response Cost</u> and <u>Direct Stuttering Reduction Strategy: Time-Out</u> (described earlier in this section); a contingency is imposed on stuttering itself, contrasted with counseling parents of stuttering children or stuttering adults.

Fluency Reinforcement Techniques. Techniques of stuttering treatment in which durations of fluency or fluent utterances of varied lengths are positively reinforced; may be used exclusively in which case, there is no contingency on rate reduction, airflow management, or other targets; may be more effective with younger children than with older children or adults; when not effective, other targets added.

- Assess the child's stuttering
- Baserate the child's stuttering frequency in the clinic
- Arrange a loosely structured treatment setting in which toys, objects, picture books, and storybooks serve as stimuli
- Evoke controlled conversational speech in a relaxed, play-oriented manner
- Select a duration-based (e.g., fluent speech sustained for 20 seconds) or topographically based (e.g., a word, phrase, or a sentence) fluency responses for reinforcement
- Describe and model fluent utterances for the child; describe and model dysfluent utterances as well
- Describe the contingency in simple terms (e.g., "I will give you a token for easy speech")
- Evoke controlled, limited utterances; use modeling
- Reinforce promptly and generously for fluent utterances or durations
- Ignore stuttering
- Increase the length of utterances or duration of utterances in gradual steps
- Train at the level of conversational speech
- Shift training to nonclinical settings
- Train parents in similar techniques and ask them to conduct home treatment sessions
- Counsel parents about the possibility of relapse and the need for booster treatment
- Follow-up and arrange for booster treatment

Fluency Shaping Techniques. A collection of somewhat varied treatment procedures for stuttering with an emphasis on teaching skills of fluency; contrasted with the Fluent Stuttering (described in this section) approach of Van Riper; the goal is natural-sounding normal fluency in everyday situations sustained over time; children are more likely to achieve this goal than adults; most adult stutterers may realize only controlled (monitored) fluency; include Fluency Reinforcement Techniques, Delayed Auditory Feedback, Regulated Breathing or Airflow Management, Gentle Phonatory Onset, Rate Reduction, and Prolonged Speech (all described in this section); little or no attention paid to feelings and attitudes; emphasis on programmed instruction and objective data collection.

Fluent Stuttering: Van Riper's Approach. An extensive, early, and influential treatment program for stuttering; also described as stuttering modification therapy; goal is to teach less abnormal, socially more acceptable stuttering, not necessarily normal fluency; contrasted with Fluency Shaping Techniques (described in this section); includes counseling and psychotherapy to change feelings and attitudes.

- Teach stuttering identification
  - teach the client to identify his or her stuttering and all associated problems including negative feelings, avoidance, word fears, and easy and difficult stutterings, with discussion, demonstration, reading, modeling, and so forth
  - teach the stutterer to identify his stuttering and associated problems in everyday speaking situations
- Desensitize to toughen the client to his or her stuttering
  - encourage the stutterer to be open and honest with his or her stuttering
  - ask the stutterer to freeze stuttering; teach the client to continue stuttering until told to stop
  - ask the client to face different audiences and stutter voluntarily to learn that most people do not react negatively, and if some do, he or she can tolerate it
- Modify stuttering by teaching more fluent, easier, and less abnormal stuttering
  - ask the client to face all feared and avoided words and begin to use them

- teach cancellation by asking the client to pause after a stuttered word and say the word again with easy and more relaxed stuttering (soft articulatory contacts and slower rate); do not ask the client to say the word fluently; ask the client to use cancellation outside the clinic
- teach pull-outs by asking the client to change stuttering in its mid-course; let the client pull himself or herself out by slowing down and using soft articulatory contacts; let the client use them outside the clinic
- teach preparatory sets by asking the client to use the techniques of modifying stuttering (easy, relaxed stuttering) as he or she anticipates difficulty on a word

Stabilize the treatment gains

- teach the client to continue to assign himself or herself speech tasks that help stabilize the use of cancellations, pull-outs, and preparatory sets
- ask the client to constantly practice the stuttering modification skills on difficult words
- reduce the frequency of client contacts
- continue to seek out difficult and previously avoided speaking situations
- reintegrate the stutterer's self-concept to include the role of a speaker who speaks mostly fluently but stutters on occasion

Van Riper, C. (1973). *The treatment of stuttering.* Englewood Cliffs, NJ: Prentice-Hall.

Gentle Phonatory Onset. Soft, easy, slow, and relaxed initiation of sounds as against harsh, abrupt, and tensed, initiation; a target behavior in the treatment of stuttering; often combined with such other target behaviors as Airflow Management, Prolonged Speech, or Rate Reduction (described in this section).

- Combine it with prolonged speech, airflow management, or both because gentle onset alone is not a sufficient treatment target
- Instruct the client on the need for gentle phonatory onset; contrast it with its opposite; point out the relationship between abrupt onset and stuttering
- Demonstrate (model) gentle and tensed/abrupt onset and show how speech may be dysfluent with the latter
- Ask the client to initiate sound softly, gently, with a relaxed posture
- Model soft and easy initiation of some vowels
- Ask the client to imitate and reinforce correct imitative productions
- Model soft articulatory contacts for consonants and relaxed production in general
- Reinforce imitative productions of soft articulatory contacts and relaxed speech production
- Model a few single-syllable words (e.g., I, bye, Hi) with soft and slow onset and ask the client to imitate
- Reinforce correct imitative productions of single syllable words
- Ask the client to produce selected simple words and phrases with gentle onset (evoked, not modeled)
- Add airflow management, prolonged speech, or both to gentle onset
- Continue treatment with the two or three targets; move through the sequence of words, phrases, controlled sentences, and conversational speech

Gradual Increase in Length and Complexity of Utterances (GILCU). One of two highly structured and programmed operant treatment approaches of the Monterey Fluency Program (described later in this section); developed and researched by B. Ryan and B. Van Kirk; involves reinforcing fluent speech starting with single-word productions and ending with conversational speech; the length and complexity of utterances are increased gradually in the intermediate steps; supported by clinical evidence.

Indirect Stuttering Treatment. Methods in which the clinician tries to manage stuttering in the client without concentrating on reducing stuttering directly; includes Counseling as Treatment for Stuttering (described earlier in this section); there is no direct work on reducing stuttering.

Integration of Stuttering Modification and Fluency Shaping. A dual approach that uses both the Stuttering Modification and Fluency Shaping Techniques (both described in this section); a procedure of treatment developed by T. Peters and B. Guitar; the dual approach is more forcefully applied to advanced stutterers than for beginning stutterers; uses a variety of handouts (e.g., understanding stuttering, how to be open about stuttering, and how to use feared words) during treatment sessions.

- Let the client understand his or her stuttering
  - be warm and friendly; describe the treatment program to the client
  - ask the client to read a brief description of stuttering, what it is, and how it develops; use the authors' handout "Understanding Your Stuttering"; answer all questions; share and reinforce the client's insights
  - catalog all aspects of the client's stuttering to give a good understanding of the problem; model stuttering, use videotapes or mirrors to demonstrate stuttering
- Reduce negative feelings and attitudes and eliminate avoidance behaviors
  - encourage the client to discuss his or her stuttering openly with family, friends, and acquaintances; use the authors' handout "Discussing Stuttering Openly" in the treatment session

   - ask the client to create a hierarchy of feared and avoided words and situations; encourage the client to use feared words and enter previously avoided speaking situations freely and frequently; use the authors' handout "Using Feared Words and Entering Feared Situations"
   - teach the client the technique of freezing or holding onto the moment of stuttering; use the authors' handout; when the client stutters, ask to continue (to repeat, prolong) until you signal to stop; teach the client to be calm while doing this
   - teach the client Voluntary Stuttering; use the authors' handout "Using Voluntary Stuttering"; explain the rationale for it; model brief, easy repetitions or prolongations for the client to imitate; take the client to naturalistic settings where the client will stutter voluntarily
- Teach fluency enhancing skills and modify the moments of stuttering
   - teach Rate Reduction in Treating Stuttering induced by DAF, Gentle Phonatory Onset (both described in this section), and Soft Articulatory Contacts; use the authors' handout, "Using Fluency Enhancing Behaviors"; fade DAF in gradual steps
   - stabilize fluency enhancing skills in conversational speech without DAF
   - initiate activities to generalize fluency to situations outside the clinic and with audience other than the clinician
   - teach easy stuttering; teach cancellation, pull-outs, and preparatory sets described under Fluent Stuttering: Van Riper' Approach (described in this section); teach the stutterer to integrate fluency enhancing skills with stuttering modification.

- initiate activities to generalize stuttering modification skills to situations outside the clinic and with other audiences
- Help maintain improvement
  - help the stutterer become his or her own clinician; use the authors' handout "Becoming Your Own Clinician"; help the client learn to design assignments to reduce fear and avoidance (e.g., voluntary stuttering in a difficult situation); encourage the client to work on stuttering and fluency everyday
  - establish long-term fluency goals; use the authors' handout; help the client set the goal of spontaneous (unmonitored) fluency whenever possible; controlled (monitored) fluency when it is important to be fluent; and controlled stuttering (mild, stuttering with which the stutterer is comfortable) when it is acceptable

Peters, T. J., & Guitar, B. (1991). *Stuttering: An integrated approach to its nature and treatment.* Baltimore, MD: Williams & Wilkins.

Metronome-Paced Speech. Speech that is regulated by the beats of a metronome; a form of treatment used for stuttering and cluttering; syllables or word initiations may be regulated; may be used to slow down or accelerate the rate of speech; documented immediate effects of reduced or eliminated stuttering, but timed, rhythmic, and unnatural sounding speech; research needed to document long-term effects; possibility of client adaptation to the beats (no more effective); Delayed Auditory Feedback (DAF) (described earlier in this section) with its similar effects, is preferred over metronome speech in the treatment of stuttering.

- Assess the client and baserate stuttering
- Select a miniaturized, battery-operated electronic metronome the client can wear like a hearing aid
- Find the client-specific beat rate that reduces or eliminates stuttering

- Have the client time the production of syllables with the beats in the early stages of treatment
- Have the client time the production of words with the beats in the later stages
- Have the client time the production of phrases and sentences as fluency increases and stabilizes
- Increase the rate of beats or vice versa, depending on the starting point
- Ask the client to initially wear the unit in all situations
- Fade the metronome beats by reducing its intensity in gradual steps
- Ask the client to wear the unit with the power turned off
- Ask the client to remove the unit
- Continue conversational therapy without the unit to stabilize fluency
- Conduct informal treatment sessions in varied nonclinical settings
- Counsel the client about the possibility of relapse and the need for Booster Treatment
- Follow-up and arrange for booster treatment

Monterey Fluency Program (MFP). A programmed operant approach to establish, transfer, and maintain fluency in persons who stutter; uses one of two specific methods: Delayed Auditory Feedback (DAF) and Gradual Increase in Length and Complexity of Utterances (GILCU); DAF is often used with older or more severe stutterers and GILCU is more frequently used with younger and less severe stutterers; contains establishment, transfer, and maintenance phases; supported by clinical evidence; developed and researched by B. Ryan and B. Van Kirk.

MFP Delayed Auditory Feedback Method

- Give an overview of the program to the client, the parents, or both; describe the role the parents or other family members will play in fluency maintenance at home

- Give a criterion test consisting of 5 minutes of reading, monologue, and conversation to baserate stuttering; measure stuttering in terms of stuttered words per minute (SW/M)
- Implement the fluency establishment program
  - teach the client to identify and measure his or her stuttering with 75% or better accuracy
  - begin by reading with the child in a slow, prolonged, and fluent manner; reinforce verbally and with tokens and require a 0 SW/M in this and the subsequent steps
  - instruct the child to read with a 250 msec DAF
  - reinforce verbally and with tokens for fluent speech and say, "stop, use your slow, prolonged speech" when the client stutters
  - decrease the DAF to 200, 150, 100, 50, and 0 msec in successive steps
  - at each step of the decreasing DAF, require a 0 SW/M (100% fluency) during a 5-minute oral reading
  - switch to monologue with 250 msec DAF when the client meets the 5-minute 0 SW/M criterion in oral reading with no DAF
  - decrease DAF in steps similar to those for oral reading
  - switch to conversational speech with 250 msec DAF when the client meets the performance criterion (0 SW/M in 5 minutes of monologue with no DAF)
  - repeat the steps to progressively decrease the DAF to zero and have the client meet the performance criterion
- Implement the fluency transfer program
  - vary the physical setting; have the client read for one minute and converse for 3 minutes with you

  in each of 5 physical settings; verbally reinforce for fluency and say "stop, speak fluently" when stuttering occurs
  - vary the audience; bring in one person (e.g., the child's classmate), then two persons, and finally three persons; each time, let the child converse with 0 SW/M
  - ask parents join you in treatment sessions; train them to conduct home reading, monologue, and conversational practice sessions
  - ask parents to conduct practice sessions at home; have the client read, engage in monologue, or conversation at home with increasing audience size as the corresponding steps are completed in the clinic
  - ask the parents to require fluent speech all the time at home and let them reinforce the child
  - transfer training to classroom; initially let the child read and converse with you in the classroom
  - eventually, have the child give an oral presentation to the class
  - have the child make telephone calls and require a 3-minute fluent conversation on the phone
  - have the child speak to strangers and require 3-minutes of fluent speech
  - instruct the child to speak fluently at all the time and in all situations
- Implement the fluency maintenance program
  - follow-up the child for 22 months; schedule follow-up sessions 2 weeks, a month, 3 months, 6 months, and 12 month intervals
  - give the criterion test at each visit (5 minutes of oral reading, monologue, and conversation with 0.5 SW/M or less)
  - if there is regression, recycle through selected steps of the treatment program
  - dismiss the child after 22 months of maintained fluency

MFP Gradual Increase in Length and Complexity of Utterances (GILCU)

- Give an overview of the program to the client, the parents, or both; describe the role the parents or other family members will play in fluency maintenance at home
- Give a criterion test consisting of 5 minutes of reading, monologue, and conversation to baserate stuttering; measure stuttering in terms of stuttered words per minute (SW/M)
- Implement the fluency establishment program
  - teach the client to identify and measure his or her stuttering with 75% or better accuracy
  - instruct the client to "read fluently"; have the client read one word fluently; reinforce with verbal praise for fluent production; say "stop, read fluently" when stuttering occurs; obtain 10 consecutively fluently read words
  - gradually increase the length of orally read responses; steps include 2, 3, 4, 5, and 6 fluent words; 1, 2, 3, and 4 fluent sentences; fluency for 30 seconds and 1, 1.5, 2, 2.5, 3, 4, and 5 minutes
  - instruct the client to "speak fluently;" ask the client to engage in monologue (first step with a nonreader); use pictures and topic ideas and other necessary stimulus procedures with the same gradually escalating steps
  - engage the child in conversation; use the same gradually escalating steps
  - reinforce fluent productions with verbal praise and tokens
  - say "stop, read fluently" or "stop, speak fluently" when the client stutters
  - model the target response when the client persists with stuttering
  - require 100 fluency (0 SW/M) at each step

- give a criterion test at the end of the establishment phase (5 minutes of reading, monologue, and conversation with 0 SW/M)
- Implement the fluency transfer program
  - use the procedure outlined earlier under *MFP Delayed Auditory Feedback Method*; skip or modify steps to suit the client (e.g., skip telephone training for a young child; select appropriate extraclinical settings for an adult)
- Implement the fluency maintenance program
  - use the procedures outlined earlier under *MFP Delayed Auditory Feedback Method*

Ryan, B., & Van Kirk, B. (1971). *Monterey fluency program.* Palo Alto, CA: Monterey Learning Systems.

Prolonged Speech. Speech produced with extended duration of speech sounds, especially vowels, and particularly those in the initial position of words; a target behavior in stuttering treatment; not a treatment procedure but the effect of treatment; induces Stutter-Free Speech; results in fluency that sounds unnatural and socially unacceptable; useful in establishing stutter-free speech; often combined with such additional targets as Natural Sounding Fluency, Airflow Management, and Gentle Phonatory Onset; a common component in many contemporary stuttering treatment programs; supported by clinical evidence, some experimentally controlled; procedurally, either DAF-induced or clinician-induced.

Prolonged Speech, DAF-Induced. Speech that is produced by prolonging speech sounds, especially the vowels, and particularly in the word-initial positions; prolongation of sounds forced by the Delayed Auditory Feedback (DAF); induces stutter-free speech that sounds fluent but unnatural and socially unacceptable; a target behavior in many stuttering treatment programs; often combined with such other targets as Airflow Management, Gentle Phonatory Onset, Normal Prosody and Natural-

Sounding Fluency; supported by clinical evidence, some experimentally controlled; clinical procedures under Delayed Auditory Feedback.

Prolonged Speech, Clinician-Induced. Speech that is produced by prolonging speech sounds, especially the vowels, and particularly in the word-initial positions; prolongation of sounds taught by clinicians without mechanical help; Instructions, Modeling, and Differential Reinforcement the most effective techniques to induce it; supported by clinical evidence, some experimentally controlled; induces stutter-free speech that sounds fluent but unnatural and socially unacceptable; a target behavior in many stuttering treatment programs; often combined with such other targets as Airflow Management, Gentle Phonatory Onset, Normal Prosody, or Natural-Sounding Fluency.

- Assess the client and baserate the stuttering rate and speech rate
- Instruct the client in producing prolonged speech and describe its need, effects, and justification
- Ask the client to prolong the vowels, and especially those at the beginning of words, phrases, grammatical clauses
- Ask the client to reduce the rate of speech throughout the utterance
- Model the prolonged speech and overall reduced speech rate
- Model words, phrases, and sentences to give the client an idea, but ask the client to imitate only what he or she can (perhaps only words); model frequently
- Reduce your own rate of speech and talk in a noticeably prolonged manner
- Reinforce the client's prolonged speech promptly and lavishly

- Tell the client to "stop" (discontinue talking) at the earliest sign of increased rate, shortened vowels, or stuttering
- Repeat modeling, especially in the early stages of treatment whenever the client fails to maintain the target behaviors or produces stuttering
- Establish stutter-free (prolonged) speech at the topographic levels of words, phrases, sentences, and spontaneous conversational speech
- Use such performance criteria as 98 or 100% fluency at each topographic level, observed for a period of time or for a certain number of responses
- Increase the length of utterance as the client meets a particular performance criterion
- Decrease the extent of prolongation gradually as the client becomes more fluent
- Ask the client to increase the rate of speech and reinforce fluency at progressively increased speech rates
- Model normal prosodic features and ask the client to imitate
- Let the client slowly and gradually return to normal rate, rhythm, and prosody while maintaining fluency
- Train family members to signal the client to speak slowly and to reinforce fluent speech in daily situations
- Train the client in Self-Control (Self-Monitoring) skills by having him or her count stutterings
- Train the client to stop and slow down every time the rate increases or stuttering returns
- Conduct informal treatment sessions in varied nonclinical settings
- Counsel the client, the family, or both about the possibility of relapse and the need for booster treatment

- Follow-up and arrange for booster treatment

Rate Reduction in Treating Stuttering. A speech rate slower than normal or below a client-specific baserate; a typical target to reduce stuttering; a component of many treatment programs; similar to prolonged speech; supported by clinical evidence; may use Delayed Auditory Feedback to induce rate reduction; appropriate with very young children especially when the DAF is omitted.

- Establish the baserate of speech rate, measured in terms of syllables per minute or words per minute
- Instruct the client in rate reduction and describe its desirable effects
- Reassure the client that a more acceptable rate is the final target of treatment
- Reduce the rate by prolonging the vowels, not by increasing pause durations between words, phrases, and sentences
- Experiment with slower rates that reduce stuttering to near zero
- Model the effective rate selected for the client
- Ask the client to imitate the slower rate in producing multisyllable words and phrases by extending the duration of syllables (not pauses)
- Use delayed auditory feedback if instructions and modeling are not effective
- Shape slower rate in multisyllable words, phrases, sentences, and conversational speech to induce Stutter-Free Speech
- Fade the excessively slow rate of speech while the client maintains stutter-free conversational speech and moves toward more Natural Sounding Fluency
- Shape the normal or near-normal rate along with Normal Prosody
- Teach Self-Control (Self-Monitoring) of rate control that the client can use when needed in everyday situations

Regulated Breathing. A direct stuttering reduction method in which the client is asked to modify breathing patterns along with the use of such other strategies as thought formulation and relaxation; some clinical evidence supports its use but the effective component of the eclectic program is not clear; developed and researched by N. Azrin and his associates; only the components, inhalation and slight exhalation before initiating phonation have been incorporated into several current treatment programs; more effective with older children and adults than with very young children.

- Ask the client to formulate thoughts before speaking
- Instruct the client to inhale and exhale a small amount of air before talking; model the target behaviors
- Ask the client to continue to exhale a little even after the last sound is produced
- Instruct the client to pause at natural speech junctures and formulate thoughts again
- Ask the client to stop soon after a stuttering occurs and relax, especially the chest muscles
- Ask the client to seek out previously avoided speaking situations
- Ask the client to practice the new method of speaking daily
- Train and ask the client to measure and record his or her stutterings in natural settings
- Train a family member in the procedure and let the person help the stutterer at home
- Maintain phone contact with the client to follow-up

Azrin, N. H., & Nunn, R. G. (1974). A rapid method of eliminating stuttering by a regulated breathing approach. *Behavior Research & Therapy, 12*, 279–286.

Replacing Stuttering with Normal Speech. A method of stuttering treatment based primarily on Delayed Auditory Feedback (DAF); includes Continuous Airflow throughout utterances and psychotherapeutic discussions; developed and researched by W. Perkins and his associates, including R. Curlee.

- Establish fluent speech
  - set the DAF at 250 msec to generate about 30 words per minute (wpm) and stutter-free speech
  - use reading or conversation, whichever is easier for the client
  - use clinician-induced prolongation if a DAF unit is not available
- Establish normal breath flow
  - begin this in the second session if not toward the end of first session
  - limit the phrase length to 3 to 8 syllables
  - teach the client to maintain airflow continuously throughout an utterance; ask the client to blend words in a smooth, continuous manner
  - teach a soft, breathy voice
  - teach gentle initiation of the initial syllable of phrases
- Establish normal prosody
  - teach normal intonation, stress pattern
  - have the client prolong stressed syllables longer and produce them louder
  - have the client produce unstressed syllables with light contacts and with less prolongation
- Shift responsibility for taking all subsequent steps to the stutterer
  - impress on the client that all subsequent steps are his or her own responsibility
  - ask the client to tape record a treatment step taken and make decisions about the degree of control, the ability to slow down when the rate accelerates, and the need to move back to an earlier step
  - ask the client to move at a comfortable speech rate
- Establish slow-normal speech in conversation
  - begin with oral reading if fluency skills have not been practiced in conversation
  - progress to slow-normal conversational speech with 250 msec DAF

- eliminate avoidance behaviors
- Incorporate psychotherapeutic discussion
  - respond affirmatively to client's positive statements about him- or herself about the speech experiences
- Establish normal speech rate
  - reduce DAF to 200 msec and increase speech rate to 45–60 wps
  - reduce DAF to 150 msec and increase speech rate to 90–120 wps
  - reduce DAF further in 50 msec intervals until a normal 150 wpm rate is achieved
  - reduce the volume of DAF
  - stabilize a "home base" rate to which the client can return when stuttering increases
- Establish normal speech without DAF
  - turn the DAF unit off
  - remove one earphone at a time
  - remove the DAF headset
- Establish a clear voice
  - if voice sounds breathy or soft, reinforce a clear, louder voice
  - ask the client to use the most effective fluency skills in everyday situations (not necessarily all those taught in the program)
- Use strategies for generalizing normal speech
  - teach the client to rate his or her fluency, rate, breath flow, prosody, and self-confidence
  - if the rating is below expected, ask the client to return to relevant shaping procedures
  - teach the client to rehearse a slow rate and breath management when he or she anticipates stuttering
  - change the therapy room and add one and then more listeners to treatment sessions
  - ask the client to face speaking situations from the least difficult to the most difficult and try to maintain normal fluency (e.g., talking on the telephone, ordering in a restaurant, talking to strangers)

- reduce the frequency of treatment sessions
- facilitate living pattern changes by encouraging the stutterer to participate in enjoyable speech activities previously not tried; ask family members to accept the newly learned normal fluency in the client

Perkins, W. H. (1973). Replacement of stuttering with normal speech: II. Clinical procedures. *Journal of Speech and Hearing Disorders, 38*, 295–303.

Shadowing. A stuttering and cluttering treatment technique in which the client, without seeing the text, repeats (shadows) everything the clinician reads from a book; the client stays a few words behind the clinician; typical effect is to reduce the frequency of stuttering; popular in the 1960s and 1970s especially in Europe; some clinician evidence suggests its effect in reducing stuttering; no research on maintenance of fluency.

- Assess the client and baserate the stuttering frequency
- Select a reading material that is suitable to the client
- Instruct the client to say everything that you read
- Give practice by reading a few sentences at a time, stopping, and reinstructing, if necessary
- Do not show the text to the client
- Read normally; do not change the rate, rhythm, or phrasing
- Tape record the client's shadowing to measure the frequency of stuttering during treatment sessions

Stutter-Free Speech. Speech of a person who stutters that contains no or few stuttering; often not the same as normally fluent speech because it may not sound natural when achieved by the use of Delayed Auditory Feedback, Rate Reduction or Prolonged Speech induced by clinicians, and by Metronome-Paced Speech; a result of initial stages of such treatment methods; needs additional procedures to make the speech sound naturally fluent and make it last over time and across situations.

Stutter-Free Speech: A Stuttering Treatment Program. A method of stuttering treatment developed and researched by G. Shames and C. Florance; uses Delayed Auditory Feedback (DAF) to induce slow, stutter-free speech; uses operant procedures to shape natural-sounding fluency.

- Teach volitional control over speech (slower rate and continuous phonation)
  - reduce the speech rate through DAF (initial delay of 250 msec)
  - train the client to produce 30 minutes of stutter-free conversational speech at progressively reduced delays of 200, 150, 100, and 50 msec to increase the speech rate
  - teach the client to stretch each word into the following word to produce continuous phonation
- Teach Self-Control (Self-Monitoring) and self-reinforcement
  - teach the client to self-monitor fluent and stuttered speech so that he or she deliberately produces an acceptable rate and continuous phonation
  - teach the client to evaluate his or her fluent and stuttered productions
  - teach the client to self-reinforce by talking without monitoring after a period of deliberately monitored speech
- Implement transfer and generalization procedures
  - develop a contract with the client that specifies speaking situations in which he or she will use the newly acquired fluency
  - ask the client to use stutter-free speech in a few situations initially and all day subsequently
  - let the client control the number and types of situations to which to transfer
  - let the client self-reinforce with unmonitored (but fluent) speech
- Replace monitored speech with unmonitored speech
  - ask the client to gradually decrease the duration for which he or she monitors fluency

- ask the client to use unmonitored but fluent speech all the time or use monitored speech only on special occasions
- Follow-up the client
  - Follow-up the client for five years

Shames, G. H., & Florence, C. L. (1980). *Stutter-free speech.* Columbus, OH: Charles E. Merrill.

Stuttering Modification. A collection of approaches to treating stuttering in which the emphasis is on changing the form of stuttering so that it is less severe and more socially and personally acceptable; the goal is not normal fluency, but less abnormality; approach exemplified by Fluent Stuttering approach of Van Riper (described earlier in this section) ; includes attempts to change attitudes and feelings; treatment sessions loosely structured; little emphasis on measurement of behaviors; contrasted with Fluency Shaping Techniques (described earlier in this section).

Stuttering Prevention: A Clinical Method. An early treatment program for children who stutter; developed by W. Strakweather and his associates; based on the Demands and Capacities Model (DCM) of fluency and stuttering; goal is to reduce demands made on the child's fluency and increase fluency capacities.

- Assess the child's capacity for fluency and the demands the child faces
- Counsel the parents

  educate the parents about stuttering, the treatment program, and prognosis; give an optimistic outlook on improvement with treatment

  change attitudes of parents by discussing their negative feelings and possible guilt

  change behaviors of parents; ask them to speak at a slower rate; ask them to use shorter, simpler sentences while speaking to the child; let them know that negative reactions and punishment can worsen stuttering; encourage polite turn taking in conversation; ask them to arrange a special talking time with the child; ask parents to demand speech less often; teach parents the direct treatment techniques

- Modify directly the child's stuttering and fluency
  - reduce the tension and struggle behaviors associated with dysfluency
  - initially, model behaviors (slower rate, less struggled word and phrase repetitions) without necessarily requiring the child to imitate them
  - later, ask the child to imitate slower rate by syllable prolongation
  - implement such fluency enhancing strategies as no interruption and no demands for verbal performance (silent periods are fine)
  - control play activities so that they are appropriate for the child's cognitive level and allows for conversation
- Include direct intervention strategies and fluency shaping procedures as found necessary
  - use gentle phonatory onset and light articulatory contacts
  - time-out contingent on struggle behaviors
  - self-correcting
- promote a level of language use that is normal for the child's age and gender
  - model a level of language use that is appropriate for the child
  - change parent's language as specified earlier
- Dismiss the child only when both the parents' and the child's behaviors have changed

Starkweather, W., Gottwald, S. R., & Halfond, M. (1990). *Stuttering prevention: A clinical method.* Englewood Cliffs, NJ: Prentice-Hall.

Vocal Feedback Device. An electronic instrument used in treating stuttering; provides delayed auditory feedback and vibrotactile sensory feedback of phonation; the unit is portable and may be worn by the client in everyday situations; used mostly as a part of Prolonged Speech, induced by Delayed Auditory Feedback.

Voluntary Stuttering. A technique of stuttering modification in which the client is asked to stutter deliberately; the goal is to reduce the fear and embarrassment associated with it and to eliminate avoidance of stuttering.

Submucous Cleft. Unexposed cleft of the hard palate, soft palate, or both because of normal mucosal covering; speech in some cases may be hypernasal.

Substitution Processes. A group of phonological processes in which one class of sounds is substituted for another; in phonological treatment, the target is to eliminate such processes; major substitution processes include:

- ***Denasalization:*** substitution of an oral consonant for a nasal consonant (e.g., /d/ for /n/)
- ***Gliding:*** substitution of a glide for a liquid (e.g., /w/ for /r/)
- ***Stopping:*** substitution of a stop for a fricative or an affricate (e.g., /p/ for /f/)
- ***Velar Fronting:*** substitution of an alveolar for a velar (e.g., /t/ for /k/)

Supraglottic Swallow Maneuver. A procedure to reduce or control aspiration while modifying swallowing behavior during the oral phase of the swallow; teaches the client to voluntarily protect the airway.

- Ask the patient to inhale and hold the breath
- Place food in the mouth
- Ask the patient to tilt the head back and swallow
- Teach the patient to cough after each swallow to clear any residual food from the pharynx

Swallow Reflex. A series of reflexive actions needed to complete the swallow; includes the reflexive elevation of the soft palate, closure of the airway, peristalsis (constriction of the pharyngeal constrictors), relaxation of the cricopharyngeal muscle to passage of food into the esophagus; often delayed in patients with dysphagia; may be triggered by stimulating the base of the anterior faucial arch.

Syndrome. A constellation of signs and symptoms that are associated with a morbid process.

Teflon™ or Collagen Injection. A medical treatment procedure for clients with paralyzed vocal cords; injected into the middle third of the cord, the two materials increase the bulk and the chances of abduction.

Terminal Response. The final response targeted in Shaping.

Time-Out (TO). Time-out from positive reinforcement; a direct response reduction procedure in which one of the following three contingencies is placed on a behavior to be reduced : (1) a brief period of no reinforcement (nonexclusion TO); (2) exclusion of the person from the stream of activity (exclusion TO), but not from the current environment; or (3) removal of the person from the current environment and placing the person in an isolated place for a brief period (Isolation TO).

Exclusion TO

- Contingent on an undesirable response, exclude the client from the current stream of activities, but not from the environment
- Let the client resume the activity at the end of the TO duration

Isolation TO

- Contingent on an undesirable response, remove the client from the current environment
- Place the client in a specially designed situation for a certain duration
- Bring the client back to the normal environment at the end of the TO duration

Nonexclusion TO

- Begin TO as soon as the client produces an undesirable response
- During TO, do not interact with client
- Ask the client not to respond for the specified duration
- At the end of the TO duration, resume interaction

Tokens. Conditioned generalized reinforcers; objects that are earned during treatment and exchanged later for back-up reinforcers.

- Always have back-up reinforcers the child can exchange the tokens for
- Let the child choose a back-up reinforcer in the beginning of each session
- Let the child understand the ratio of tokens to a back-up reinforcer
- Set a low ratio in the beginning and gradually raise the number of tokens needed to receive the back-up

Tongue Thrust. A deviant swallow in which the tongue is pushed forward against the central incisors.

Topic Initiation. A pragmatic language skill to initiate conversation on a topic; a frequent language intervention target; procedures described under Language Disorders in Children; Treatment of Language Disorders: Specific Techniques or Programs.

Topic Maintenance. A pragmatic language skill to maintain conversation for socially acceptable time periods; a frequent language intervention target; procedures described under Language Disorders in Children: Treatment of Language Disorders: Specific Techniques or Programs.

Topographic Sequence of Treatment. Sequencing treatment based on response complexity.

- Begin treatment with simpler topographic levels (word, phrases)
- Increase the topographic complexity in gradual steps (sentences, conversational speech)

Topography. Description of natural and physical properties of an object or event; topographic aspects of skills refer to their physical form or shape including how complex they are, and how they appear, sound, and feel.

Total Communication. The simultaneous use of multiple modes of expression to enhance communication; includes speech, gestures, informal and formal (e.g., American Sign Language and AMER-IND) signs, and facial expressions.

Tracheoesophageal Fistulization/Puncture (TEF/TEP). A surgical procedure that helps laryngectomy patients to produce alaryngeal speech with the help of a voice prosthesis; the tracheal wall is punctured to create a small tunnel into the esophagus; the puncture acts as a shunt to allow air into the esophagus through a Voice Prosthesis inserted into the opening; air goes up through the P-E Segment and results in the production of sound.

Andrews, M. L. (1995). *Manual of voice treatment: Pediatrics to geriatrics*. San Diego, CA: Singular Publishing Group.

Casper, J. K., & Colton, R. H. (1993). *Clinical manual for laryngectomy and head and neck cancer rehabilitation*. San Diego, CA: Singular Publishing Group.

Traditional Orthography. Written natural language; a normal form of communication; a method of nonvocal communication for the speechless; used in teaching Augmentative Communication Gestural-Assisted (aided).

Training Broad. An approach to treating articulation disorders in which several sounds are treated simultaneously; practice, limited on any one sound, is given over a broad range of sounds. Contrasted with Training Deep.

Training Criterion. A rule that specifies when an exemplar or a target skill has met a targeted performance level; a 90% correct response rate is an often accepted training criterion.

- Specify a training criterion in measurable terms (e.g., 9 out of 10 correct responses)
- Continue training until that criterion is met
- Probe when the training criterion is met
- If the probe criterion is not met, resume training

Training Deep. An approach to treating articulation disorders in which one or a few sounds are trained intensively; other sounds are selected for training only when the child has mastered the initial targets; contrasted with Training Broad.

Training Sessions in Natural Environments. Part of extraclinical training strategy used to promote maintenance.

- Initially, hold training in varied settings in and around the clinic
- Next, hold informal training sessions in nonclinical settings
- Train parents to hold training sessions at home
- Take the client to such natural setting as shopping centers and restaurants
- Let the training in natural settings be less conspicuous, involving mostly conversational speech
- Deliver reinforcers and corrective feedback in a subtle manner

Traumatic Brain Injury (TBI). An injury to the brain; may be Penetrating (Open-Head) Injury or Nonpenetrating (Closed-Head) Injury; major symptoms include restlessness, irritation, disorientation to time and place, disorganized and inconsistent responses; impaired memory, attention, reasoning, drawing, naming, and repetition; also known as craniocerebral trauma; immediate concern is medical; long-term concern is rehabilitation.

Treatment of Traumatic Brain Injury: General Principles

- Treatment and rehabilitation are long-term
- Different kinds of therapeutic activities are scheduled at different stages of recovery from TBI (acute, postacute, outpatient, and long-term)
- It is important to work with the family and medical and rehabilitation staff from the beginning
- Speech-language pathologists are members of rehabilitation teams that include different professionals
- Communication training gains momentum as the patient recovers from the initial effects of TBI
- Physical rehabilitation is an important aspect of treatment
- The goal of treatment is functional communication
- Initial treatment sessions are brief and frequent

- Subsequent treatment may be longer and less frequent
- Compensatory strategies may be necessary for most clients
- Treatment sessions need to be structured and distraction-free in the beginning
- Treatment tasks should be carefully sequenced

Traumatic Brain Injury, Treatment Procedures

Treatment During the Initial Stage

- Simplify activities and routines
- Decrease variability in activities and stimulation
- Induce consistency in staff care and stimuli
- Improve the client's orientation and attention to surroundings
  - arrange familiar cues by pasting familiar pictures, posters, and objects
  - play favorite music
  - post written signs about the daily routines
  - ask questions about time, place, and people; prompt correct responses
  - frequently model any response you expect from the client
  - simplify all demands so that the client experiences successes
  - use tangible reinforcers
  - keep the treatment sessions brief
  - prompt and assist the client to engage in self-care activities
  - gradually reduce the amount of physical help offered
  - have the client participate in group treatment sessions as soon as it is practical
  - place behavioral contingencies on appropriate behaviors
  - shape desired targets
- Pair gestures with verbal explanations
- Use auditory stimulation as the chief method of input
- Do not overstimulate
- Use brightly colored objects and pictures in treatment
- Start with strong cues and fade later

- Use graphs and charts to show the patient relationships between objects
- Relate the information to experiences that have occurred in the patient's life
- Teach the patient to respond with *yes* or *no*
- Introduce familiar sounds from the patient's home (e.g., dog bark)
- Use familiar odors to reorient patient to previously identifiable smells
- Gain the patient's attention
- Reduce complexity and rate of speech if necessary
- Use statements instead of questions when initially communicating with the patient
- Prompt, gesture, and use verbal instructions to help the patient comprehend
- Allow the patient time to listen to instructions
- Use sentence completion tasks for patients with initiation or inhibition difficulties
- Place contingencies on appropriate behaviors

Treatment During the Intermediate Stage

- Continue to place contingencies on target behaviors
- Establish more complex routines
- Target more complex communicative skills for treatment
- Continue to provide additional stimuli as needed (written instructions, alarms, posters, verbal reminders of activities and appointments)
- Repeat treatment trials
- Improve selective attention and comprehension by asking the patient to:
  - match pictures to sentences
  - follow spoken instructions
  - retell a message to another person
  - answer simple questions
- Work closely with health care workers; teach them to
  - recognize the client's problems
  - respond promptly to positive changes in communication skills

- provide additional stimuli as needed
- Work with family members; teach them to
  - prompt the client when there is hesitation
  - model appropriate behaviors
  - reinforce the behaviors naturally and sustain those behaviors
- Increase awareness of deficits
  - use simple explanations to describe the problem to the patient
  - give contingent feedback on problem behaviors
  - use group therapy to allow the patient to see that others have similar problems
- Continue group treatment to have peer modeling, monitoring, and self-awareness of problems
- Begin to diminish special stimuli and reminders as performance improves toward the end of the intermediate stage
- Begin to teach Self-Control (Self-Monitoring) skills
- Begin to teach compensatory skills

Treatment During the Late Stage

- Train more complex activities that enhance independence
- Further diminish special stimuli (posters, verbal reminders, written instructions) that control behaviors
- Continue to use shaping, modeling, prompting, and manual guidance to enhance correct responses and to reduce the probability of errors
- Treat Motor Speech Disorders
- Teach Self-Control (Self-Monitoring) skills; teach the client to
  - keep possessions in specific places
  - count his or her own errors in treatment
  - self-correct errors
  - use self-cueing strategies (pausing after an error)
- Teach compensatory strategies if necessary, by teaching patients to:

- break down tasks into smaller, more manageable components
- request information relative to time, date, and so forth
- rehearse important information
- write down instructions, appointments, and so forth
- ask for written instructions from people
- use active instead of passive cues (an alarm instead of a reminder in a diary)

- Teach organizational strategies by teaching the patient to:
  - separate relevant from irrelevant material
  - summarize, highlight, and take notes
  - self-monitor
- Ask patients to copy symbols, letters, and words that commonly occur in their surroundings (e.g., signs which read, "no drinking, smoking, and eating")
- Develop a core vocabulary that the patient is likely to use every day
- Teach the patient to recognize letters, syllables, words, phrases, and sentences

Beukelman, D. R., & Yorkston, K. M. (1991). *Communication disorders following traumatic brain injury: Management of cognitive, language, and motor impairments*. Austin, TX: Pro-Ed.

Bilger, E. D. (Ed.). (1990). *Traumatic brain injury*. Austin, TX: Pro-Ed.

Hegde, M. N. (1994). *A coursebook on aphasia and other neurogenic language disorders*. San Diego, CA: Singular Publishing Group.

Brookshire, R. H. (1992). *An introduction to neurogenic communication disorders*. St. Louis, MO: Mosby Year Book.

Ylvisaker, M. (1985). *Head injury rehabilitation: Children and adolescents*. Austin, TX: Pro-Ed.

Traumatic Brain Injury (TBI) in Children. Cerebral injury due to external force; may be Penetrating (Open-Head) Injury or Nonpenetrating (Closed-Head) Injury; communicative disorders are a common consequence of TBI; treatment procedures described under Traumatic Brain Injury, Treatment and many described under Language Disorders in Children are generally applicable with the following special considerations:

- Assess residual language and communication difficulties
- Design a treatment program that will address the residual deficits
- Consider the child's social and family communication needs
- Work closely with educators and teach skills that help academic achievement:
  - discuss the child's needs with other school professionals including teachers, educational psychologists, reading specialists, and others
  - develop a treatment plan that addresses the concerns of educators
  - target functional communication skills necessary for classroom adjustment
  - target specific academic terms for language intervention
  - integrate reading and writing into your treatment tasks
- Work with the teacher to help her with classroom communication and general behavior; suggest to the teacher that she should
  - simplify the academic tasks for the child
  - shape difficult tasks
  - use simpler language spoken in slower rate
  - limit distractions in the classroom
  - keep the classroom situation organized with little variation
  - use gestures and signs along with verbal expressions
  - repeat instructions, give written instructions
  - ask the child to repeat her instructions
  - make sure that the child takes adequate notes
  - encourage the child to request help and promptly reinforce such attempts
  - accept any mode of expression initially but should expect more refined verbal communication eventually
- Keep the teacher and other educators serving the child informed of your treatment targets, general procedures, and outcome

- Ask other professionals to reinforce the skills you have taught
- Work closely with family members; train them to support the child's communicative attempts by positive reinforcement
- Develop a home treatment program and train parents in its implementation

Bilger, E. D. (Ed.). (1990). *Traumatic brain injury*. Austin, TX: Pro-Ed.

Ylvisaker, M. (1985). *Head injury rehabilitation: Children and adolescents*. Austin, TX: Pro-Ed.

Mira, M. P., Tucker, B. F., & Tyler, J. S. (1992). *Traumatic brain injury in children and adolescents*. Austin, TX: Pro-Ed.

Treatment. Application of a variable that can induce changes; use of any effective procedure in teaching new communicative skills; behaviorally, management of contingent relations between antecedents, responses, and consequences; conceptually, a rearrangement of communicative relationships between a speaker and his or her listener.

Treatment of Communicative Disorders: General Procedures That Apply Across Disorders. Common procedures used in treating most if not all disorders of communication; modified to suit the individual client, his or her specific problems, the specific target behaviors, and in light of the performance data.

- Assess the client
  - determine the diagnosis
  - describe the strengths and limitations of the client
  - describe the client's current level of communicative performance
- Evaluate the client's family constellation
  - describe the family support and resources
  - describe the social, educational or occupational demands made on the client
- Select functional, client-specific target behaviors
  - select behaviors that, when treated, will have the greatest effects on the client's communication in social situations
  - select both the short- and long-term targets

- define the dismissal criterion
- Establish the pretreatment measures or baselines of target behaviors
  - select stimuli for evoking the target behaviors
  - repeat the measures to establish reliability
  - use the Baseline Evoked Trials and Baseline Modeled Trials
  - take an extended conversational speech sample
  - obtain home sample if possible
- Design a flexible therapeutic environment
  - use the degree of control and structure that is necessary
  - gradually, loosen the structure to make the treatment environment more like the client's everyday environment
- Write a treatment program; specify
  - the target behaviors
  - treatment procedures
  - reinforcing or feedback procedures
  - Criteria for Making Clinical Decisions (moving from one level of treatment to another)
  - Probe procedure
  - maintenance procedure
  - follow-up
  - booster treatment
- Implement the treatment program
  - use objects, pictures, demonstrated actions, and so forth to evoke the target behaviors
  - give instructions, demonstrations, explanations
  - model the target responses
  - prompt the target responses
  - use manual guidance to assist the client in producing the target responses
  - shape the responses
  - fade the special stimuli including pictures, objects, modeling, prompts, and manual guidance
  - give prompt positive feedback to the client; use natural reinforcers; if you used tangible reinforcers, fade them; decrease the amount of feedback given

- give prompt corrective feedback to the client; say "no" or "wrong"; use other procedures as found appropriate (time-out, response cost)
- start treatment at a simpler level; however, if the client can perform at a higher level, do not use the lower level
- probe for generalized production as often as necessary
- shift treatment, in progressive steps, to more complex levels as the client meets the probe criterion
- always train the target behaviors in conversational speech with natural consequences

- Implement the maintenance program
  - train family members, teachers, friends, and professional caregivers in supporting the client's communicative behaviors
  - teach them to evoke the target behaviors and reinforce the client naturally
  - shift training to nonclinical settings
  - invite other persons to treatment sessions
  - have family members conduct informal treatment sessions at home
  - have teachers focus on the target skills you teach and integrate those skills in the classroom work
  - tech the client to self-monitor his or her errors and target behaviors
  - teach the client to count his or her relevant behaviors
  - teach the client to self-correct mistakes
  - teach the client to cue him- or herself
  - teach the client to pause soon after an error response is produced
  - dismiss the client when responses are reliably produced in natural settings
- Follow-up the client
  - set up a schedule for follow-up
- follow-up a client for a duration necessary to show maintenance
  - take a conversational speech sample during follow-up sessions

  - measure the production of relevant communicative skills
  - recommend booster treatment if the skills have deteriorated
- Arrange for booster treatment
  - give the same or better treatment
  - probe the response rates
  - schedule the next follow-up if necessary

Hegde, M. N. (1993). *Treatment procedures in communicative disorders* (2nd ed.). Austin, TX: Pro-Ed.

Treatment of Communicative Disorders: A General Sequence that Applies Across Disorders. Step-wise progression of treatment used in treating disorders of communication; the sequence may be based on response topography, response modes, multiple targets, training and maintenance, and response consequences.

- Sequence and simplify the target behaviors topographically
  - syllables or words
  - phrases
  - sentences that are imitated or otherwise controlled
  - sentences that are more spontaneously produced
  - sentences that are fully spontaneously produced
  - conversational speech
  - begin treatment at the simplest level that is necessary for the client; do not routinely start training at the syllable or word level; experiment to see if the client can manage at a higher level
- Sequence the response modes
- Begin treatment with imitation as the initial response mode if necessary
  - move to evoked responses
- Sequence the multiple targets
  - teach the most useful behaviors earlier than the less useful ones
  - teach the simpler behaviors earlier than the more complex behaviors
  - teach first behaviors that are building blocks for other behaviors

- when one target behavior reaches the probe criterion, select another behavior or shift training to more complex level on the behavior under training
- Sequence training and maintenance strategies
  - initially establish the behavior under structured clinical situations
  - loosen the structure gradually and make treatment conditions more similar to natural conditions
  - shift treatment to more natural conditions in and around the clinic
  - shift training to natural conditions away from the clinic
  - shift training to home situations, but do this as soon as possible (do not wait until the last stage of training)
- Sequence response consequences or feedback variations
  - give more frequent and consistent feedback in the beginning
  - reduce the amount of feedback as the learning stabilizes
  - give tangible reinforcers if necessary and only in the beginning
  - shift to social and more natural reinforcers
  - train others to give natural feedback in naturalistic settings

Hegde, M. N. (1993). *Treatment procedures in communicative disorders* (2nd ed.). Austin, TX: Pro-Ed.

Treatment of Communicative Disorders: Procedural Modifications. Changes made in treatment procedures because of their ineffectiveness or less than optimum effectiveness; modifications may be made in antecedents, responses, and consequences; treatment procedures, not principles, are modified; based on performance data.

- Modification of antecedents
  - change stimuli that are ineffective in evoking the target responses
  - shift from pictures to objects
  - shift from line drawings to photographs
  - shift from abstract to concrete stimuli
  - shift from pictorial representation to enacted stimuli
  - discard clinical stimuli in favor of stimuli from the client's home

- model if evoking is not effective
- prompt if evoking is not effective
- provide manual guidance (physical assistance to execute a response) if the evoking techniques are not effective
- give instructions and repeat them
- ask effective, common questions to evoke the responses
- rephrase ineffective questions

- Modification of responses
  - simplify the response if a more complex topographic feature is ineffective (too difficult)
  - if the target is not produced in sentences, shift downward in progressive steps
  - abandon training on a behavior that is too difficult for the client in favor of one that is easier; use the baseline data for guidance
  - abandon training on a behavior that is not imitated in favor of the one that is
  - return to abandoned behaviors at later date; shape them in small steps
- Modification of consequences
  - use the operational definition of consequences; events should increase behaviors to be called reinforcers; decrease to be called punishers or corrective
  - change consequating events that do not increase behaviors
  - change consequating events that do not decrease behaviors
  - use primary reinforcers if social consequences do not reinforce
  - shift back to social reinforcers after the behaviors are established
  - use tokens backed up by a variety of reinforcers if other forms fail
  - use biofeedback if other forms fail

Hegde, M. N. (1993). *Treatment procedures in communicative disorders* (2nd ed.). Austin, TX: Pro-Ed.

Treatment Evaluation. Testing the immediate effects and long-term efficacy of treatment procedures by controlled experimental analysis; an important criterion in treatment selection; group or single-subject experimental designs are essential in evaluating treatment effects and efficacy.

- Search the literature to see if a treatment method has been evaluated through controlled experimentation; ask the following questions:
  - has it been evaluated with a control and experimental group to show that the treatment is better than no treatment? If not
  - has it been evaluated with one of the single-subject experimental designs?
  - has the advocate ruled-out the influence of such extraneous variables as maturation and events in the life of the clients and the work of other persons including family members?
  - has the technique been shown to be effective when used by different clinicians, in different professional settings, and with different and diverse clients?
  - has the technique been shown to produce lasting effects?
- If the answer to these questions is no, select another procedure that has received experimental evaluation; select the procedure for your own experimental evaluation; or use the procedure with caution and collect systematic data.

Treatment Evoked Trials. Structured and temporally separated opportunities for the client to produce a target response in the absence of clinician's modeling; useful in establishing target behaviors, especially with clients who perform better under a highly structured treatment session.

- Place stimulus item in front of client or demonstrate an action
- Ask the relevant predetermined question
- Wait a few seconds for client to respond
- If the response is correct, reinforce the client
- If the response is incorrect, give corrective feedback
- Record the response on the recording sheet
- Remove stimulus item

- Wait 2–3 seconds to signify end of trial
- Begin the next trial
- Calculate the percent correct response rate

Treatment Modeled Trials. Structured and temporally separated opportunities for the client to produce a target response when the clinician models the response for the client to imitate.

- Place a stimulus item in front of the client or demonstrate an action
- Ask the predetermined question
- Immediately model the correct response
- If the response is correct, reinforce the client
- If the response is incorrect, give corrective feedback
- Wait a few seconds for client to respond
- Record the response on the recording sheet
- Remove the stimulus item
- Wait 2–3 seconds to signify end of trial
- Calculate the percent correct response rate

Treatment Selection Criteria. General guidelines on selecting treatment procedures; select procedures according to the following criteria; note that the criteria are hierarchically arranged; a higher criterion is more stringent, more difficult to meet, although more preferable than a lower criterion.

- Select treatment procedures that have been evaluated in controlled experiments and are shown to have generality through Replication; see Treatment Evaluation
- Select treatment procedures that have been evaluated in controlled experiments
- Select treatment procedures that have been evaluated at least through multiple case studies
- Select treatment procedures that have been shown to be effective at least in a case study
- Select treatment procedures that are logically consistent, theoretically sound, and based on solid clinical practice;

treat such procedures as experimental; collect data on their effects in your client; discard them if they are not effective
- Reject procedures based solely on opinions, speculation, questionable theories, bandwagon, popularity, and those which their long-time advocates themselves have never taken time to experimentally evaluate
- Select untested procedures only for experimental evaluation, not routine clinical practice

Treatment Targets. Skills or behaviors that are taught to clients during treatment.
- Select treatment targets after a thorough assessment
- Select functional targets that are useful to the client
- Select targets that are linguistically and culturally appropriate to the client
- Select skills that can make an immediate and socially significant difference in the communicative skills of the client
- Select behaviors that serve as building blocks for more complex functional skills

Treatment or Teaching Versus Stimulation. See Stimulation Versus Treatment or Teaching.

Treatment Variables. Technical operations performed by the clinician to create, increase, or decrease behaviors; these include:
- Antecedents or stimuli used in treatment, including modeling, instructions, demonstrations, manual guidance, pictures, objects, recreated events, storytelling (by the clinician), topics of conversation, and so forth
- Consequences or feedback the clinician gives, including verbal praise, tokens, tangible reinforcers, opportunities to indulge in various activities, privileges offered by parents, and so forth

Tremor. A pattern of shaking, defined as an involuntary rhythmical movement of small amplitude.

Trials. Measurable opportunities to produce a response; may be more or less structured; include Baseline Evoked Trials, Baseline Modeled Trials, Treatment Evoked Trials, and Treatment Modeled Trials.

Unconditioned Reinforcers. The same as Primary Reinforcers.

Unilateral Upper Motor Neuron Dysarthria. A type of motor speech disorder; its neuropathology is damage to the upper motor neurons that supply cranial and spinal nerves involved in speech production; the dominant speech problem is imprecise production of consonants; select appropriate treatment targets and procedures described under Dysarthria, Treatment; in addition, consider the following that apply especially to unilateral upper motor neuron dysarthria:

- Use behavioral methods to improve rate, prosody, and articulation
- Teach compensatory behaviors
- Use a mirror to monitor drooling

Duffy, J. R. (1995). *Motor speech disorders.* St. Louis, MO: C.V. Mosby.

Johns, D. F. (Ed.). (1985). *Clinical management of neurogenic communicative disorders.* Boston: Little, Brown.

Yorkston, K. M., Beukelman, D. R., & Bell, K. R. (1988). *Clinical management of dysarthric speakers.* Austin, TX: Pro-Ed.

Unilateral Vocal Fold Paralysis. Paralysis of one of the two vocal folds.

Validity. The degree to which a measuring instrument measures what it purports to measure; treatment procedures may have Logical Validity, Empirical Validity, or both; procedures that have empirical validity are preferable to those with only logical validity.

Verbal Corrective Feedback. A method to reduce incorrect responses in treatment; feedback is presented soon after an incorrect response is made; includes such verbal feedback as "No," "Wrong," or "Not correct"; often combined with Nonverbal Corrective Feedback.

Verbal Stimulus Generalization. Production of unreinforced responses when untrained verbal stimuli are presented; measured on a Probe.

- Present the same physical stimulus as used in training (e.g., the picture of two books used in teaching an exemplar of the plural morpheme)
- Ask a question other than the one used in training to evoke the response (e.g., if you asked "What do you see?" on training trials, ask "What are these?" on these probe trials)
- Do not model and do not provide any response consequences
- Record the response
- Present at least 10 trials, each involving a different picture and probe question (different from the training question)

Variable Interval Schedule (VI). An intermittent reinforcement schedule in which the time duration between reinforcers is varied around an average; not as applicable as the Fixed Interval or Variable Ratio Schedules in the treatment of communicative disorders; difficult to use in routine clinical work; efficient with an electronic programming equipment.

Variable Ratio Schedule (VR). An intermittent reinforcement schedule in which the number of responses needed to earn a reinforcer is varied around an average.

- Vary the number of responses required for reinforcement from one occasion to the other

Ventricular Dysphonia. A voice disorder resulting from the use of the ventricular (false) vocal folds for phonation; possibly because the true folds have some pathology; characterized by low pitch, monotone, decreased loudness, Harshness, and arrhythmic voicing.

- Teach the client to take a prolonged inhalation through open mouth and sustained exhalation without phonation
- Teach the client Inhalation Phonation (this is usually true cord phonation)
- Ask the client to produce inhalation phonation-exhalation phonation on the same breath
- Ask the client to produce a matching exhalation phonation
- Have the client practice exhalation phonation
- Teach the client to vary the pitch
- Fade inhalation-exhalation; stabilize normal phonation in conversational speech

Vocally Abusive Behaviors. A variety of behaviors that negatively affect the laryngeal mechanism and result in voice disorders; intervention described under Voice Disorders; Treatment of Vocally Abusive Behaviors; include the following:

- Excessive talking or singing
- Excessively loud talking or singing
- Yelling, cheering, and screaming
- Excessive and chronic coughing and throat clearing
- Constant talking or singing during episodes of allergy and upper respiratory infection
- Smoking
- Constant talking in noisy environments
- Speaking with hard glottal attack
- Singing or talking at the upper or lower end of the pitch range
- Excessive crying or laughing

Vocal Fold Paralysis. Unilateral or bilateral paralysis of the folds that results in fixated fold or folds; unilateral more common; often due to trauma or accidental cutting of the recurrent laryngeal nerve; results in aphonia or dysphonia; Teflon[R] or collagen may be injected into the paralyzed fold to make it bulge and help approximate.

- Consider teaching the client the use of an electronic larynx
- Provide voice therapy designed to improve loudness through respiratory control

Vocal Hyperfunction. Vocally abusive behaviors that cause nodules, polyps, and associated voice disorders; specifically, speaking with excessive muscular effort and force.

- Assess the disorder to find out the specific kinds of vocally abusive behaviors the client exhibits
- Reduce the vocally abusive behaviors
- Experiment with different Specific Normal Voice Facilitating Techniques (described under Voice Disorders) to promote normal or vastly improved voice
- Use those techniques to teach the client the more relaxed and normal voice production

Vocal Nodules. Benign lesions of the vocal folds; generally bilateral; found in the anterior one-third and posterior two-thirds of the true vocal folds; symptoms may include Hoarseness, Harshness, periodic Aphonia, frequent throat clearing, Hard Glottal Attacks, tension, and a dry vocal tract; result of vocal abuse.

- Reduce Vocally Abusive Behaviors
- Increase the breath support for speech
- Reduce vocal intensity
- Use Specific Normal Voice Facilitation Techniques (described under Voice Disorders) to teach the client to produce healthy voice

Voice Disorders. Various disorders of communication related to faulty, abnormal, or inappropriate phonation, loudness, pitch, and resonance; causes include vocally abusive behaviors, trauma to the laryngeal mechanism, and physical diseases; many treated both medically and behaviorally; some only medically; and others only behaviorally.

Voice Disorders of Loudness. Socially inappropriate voice that is too loud or soft.

Voice Disorders of Pitch. Voice characterized by inappropriate pitch; speech at the low end of one's pitch range which requires too much effort and force; or speech at the high end of the range which causes fatigue.

Voice Disorders of Phonation. Voice problems that result from vocal folds that are altered by vocally abusive behaviors, trauma, or diseases; voice that is characterized by varying degrees of breathiness, hoarseness, harshness, and pitch and loudness deviations.

Voice Disorders of Phonation: Abuse-Based. Such voice problems as hoarseness, breathiness, and harshness that result from vocal abuse which often causes physical changes in the vocal cords

Voice Disorders of Phonation: Physically-Based. Such voice problems as hoarseness, breathiness, and harshness that result from physical diseases; varied voice problems associated with laryngeal trauma.

Voice Disorders of Resonance. Voice characterized by inappropriate resonance including Hypernasality and Hyponasality.

Treatment of Voice Disorders: General Principles

- Consider the goal of voice therapy as normal sounding voice with little or no effort and tension
- Make a thorough evaluation of the voice disorder
- Make an assessment of the client's vocally abusive behaviors at home and in other natural settings
- Maintain a cooperative working relationship with a laryngologist
- Be knowledgeable about laryngeal surgical procedures, medication, and their effects on and interactions with voice treatment methods
- Always have a medical evaluation completed before starting voice therapy

- Have periodic medical examination during voice therapy
- Combine, in most cases, techniques designed to reduce vocally abusive behaviors with those that facilitate efficient and normal voice production
- Individualize the facilitating techniques because what works with one client may not work with another
- The first priority in treating voice disorders in most children is to reduce vocally abusive behaviors and the second priority is to teach optimal vocal behaviors
- Generally, the first priority in treating voice disorders in adults is to teach optimal vocal behaviors and the second priority is to reduce vocally abusive behaviors
- Work closely with parents and others to help reduce vocally abusive behaviors and to reinforce healthy vocal behaviors
- Establish baselines of vocally abusive behaviors and the frequency of abnormal voice productions in and outside the clinic

Treatment of Disorders of Loudness and Pitch

General Procedures

- Rule-out hearing loss before you attempt modification of loudness
- Establish the baseline loudness or pitch of the client
- Discuss the problem with older children and adults
- Give feedback on the client's problematic loudness or pitch by tape-recorded samples of the client's speech and your speech for comparison
- Reinforce a range of acceptable loudness and pitch variations because vocal intensity and pitch vary across speaking situations
- Role play different speaking situations and reinforce appropriate loudness and pitch levels
- Use such biofeedback instruments as the Vocal Loudness Indicator, Visi-Pitch™, and any available computer programs for voice therapy to increase shape the desired loudness and vocal pitch
- Promote maintenance of the new vocal loudness and pitch in natural settings by shifting treatment to such

settings and by teaching Self-Control (Self-Monitoring) skills

Treatment of Excessively Loud Voice

Shape progressively softer voice in a client with too loud voice:

- Model the desired loudness level
- With or without biofeedback instruments, begin training by reducing the loudness level; reinforce progressively softer voice until the level is acceptable

Treatment of Excessively Soft Voice

Shape progressively louder voice in a client with too soft voice:

- With or without biofeedback instruments, begin training by increasing the loudness level
- Experiment with different pitch levels to see if a change in pitch results in increased loudness; if so, reinforce the client for speaking at that pitch
- Use the Pushing Approach (described later in this section under Specific Normal Voice Facilitating Techniques) only if instruction, modeling, and biofeedback fail
- Model the desired loudness frequently
- Reinforce progressively louder voice until the level is acceptable

Treatment of Pitch Disorders

Treatment to Raise the Baseline Pitch

- Instruct the client on pitch, its variations, and acceptable range
- Model different levels of pitch for the client
- Experiment with the client to see if he or she can produce a desirable pitch even if briefly
- Tape record the client's desirable pitch and use it as a model for self-imitation
- Provide also a live model or a mechanical model on such computerized instruments as Visi-Pitch™, B & K Real-Time Frequency Analyzer™
- Use such instruments to give immediate feedback during training trials or durations

- Begin treatment with single words, preferably those that begin with vowels; have the client produce them with the desirable pitch
- Increase the response complexity by moving to words, phrases, sentences, and conversational speech
- Use oral reading to stabilize the desired pitch
- Provide mechanical as well as live social reinforcers
- Implement a maintenance program by conducting informal treatment in nonclinical settings
- Encourage the client to use the new pitch in all speaking situations
- Train family members, teachers, and others to prompt the client to use the new pitch and reinforce when he or she does

Treatment to Lower the Baseline Pitch

- Use the same procedures used for raising the pitch except for setting a lower pitch as the target
- Lower the pitch in carefully graded steps, if necessary

Treatment of Disorders of Phonation

Treatment of Abuse-Based Disorders of Phonation

- Make an assessment of vocally abusive behaviors
- Eliminate or reduce vocally abusive behaviors; use procedures described later in this section
- Refer the client for periodic medical examination
- Make periodic assessment of voice if and when the medical or surgical treatment is repeated
- Follow-up the client to ensure that vocally appropriate behaviors are maintained

Treatment of Physically Based Disorders of Phonation

- Refer the client with voice problems to a medical specialist to have an assessment of the physical bases of the problems
- Work closely with the medical professionals who treat the physical diseases or laryngeal trauma
- Provide voice therapy following medical or surgical treatment if found necessary and useful

- Tailor treatment to the residual problem; consider teaching proper and optimal use of voice and appropriate loudness and pitch.
- Treat patients with Laryngectomy with appropriate communication rehabilitation techniques
- Make periodic assessment of voice if and when surgical treatments are repeated

Treatment of Disorders of Resonance

General Principles

- Make an assessment of the specific resonance problem: Hypernasality or Hyponasality.
- Rule out the presence of cleft palate or congenital palatopharyngeal incompetence as the source of resonance problems; do not offer behavioral voice therapy for such cases unless the organic problems are eliminated or significantly improved by surgical or prosthetic means and clients are now good candidates for voice therapy
  - work with the prosthodontist in the client-specific fabrication of a prosthetic device
  - assess speech before and after surgical and prosthetic treatment
- Use biofeedback instruments to monitor and reinforce appropriate oral and nasal resonance

Treatment of Hypernasality

- Assess Hypernasality and treat it only when there is adequate or at least marginal velopharyngeal adequacy and the disorder needs behavioral management
- Use treatment procedures described under Hypernasality

Treatment of Hyponasality

- Assess Hyponasality and treat it only when it is clear that too broad a pharyngeal flap or too big an obturator bulb is not the source of reduced nasality
- Be aware that very few persons exhibit hyponasality with no physical basis

- Use treatment procedures described under Hyponasality

Treatment of Vocally Abusive Behaviors

- Make a thorough assessment of vocally abusive behaviors
- Explain to the client and the family the harmful results of vocally abusive behaviors the client exhibits
- Ask the client to measure his or her vocally abusive behaviors for a few days and graph their frequency on a daily basis to establish the baselines of vocally abusive behaviors in natural settings
- Ask the parents of young children to count and graph vocally abusive behaviors on a daily basis
- Design and implement a program to reduce the vocally abusive behaviors
  - use such treatment techniques as Changing Criterion to shape down the frequency of vocally abusive behaviors
  - ask the client, parent, a spouse, teacher, or a friend to help establish the reliability of measures of vocally abusive behaviors
  - in progressive steps, decrease the frequency of specified vocally abusive behaviors (e.g., the first week after a baseline of 10 episodes of screaming by a child, a criterion of 7 episodes may be held; in following weeks, the number is systematically reduced finally to zero; in case of a child who talks too much, periods of silence may be required and increased in frequency, duration, or both)
  - implement a token system for reinforcing the client for having met the criterion
- During the treatment sessions, modify specific vocally abusive behaviors by teaching the client to:
  initiate sounds softly
  - speak with optimum pitch
  - speak at an appropriate loudness
  - reduce the frequency of coughing or throat clearing

- breathe through the nose
- use an easy, relaxed breathing pattern when speaking
- speak with relaxed speech muscles
- open mouth more widely during talking

- Measure the effects of the program to document the desirable changes in the voice disorder being treated
- Follow-up the client and arrange for booster treatment

Andrews, M. L. (1995). *Manual of voice treatment: Pediatrics through geriatrics*. San Diego, CA: Singular Publishing Group.

Boone, D. R., & McFarlane, S. C. (1988). *The voice and voice therapy* (4th ed.). Englewood Cliffs, NJ: Prentice Hall.

Prater, R. J., & Swift, R. W. (1984). *Manual of voice therapy*. Austin, TX: Pro-Ed.

Specific Normal Voice Facilitating Techniques. A collection of procedures used in voice therapy; most are based on clinical experience; little or no controlled experimental evidence to demonstrate their effectiveness and efficacy; need more research data.

Altered Tongue Position. Manipulating tongue position in the oral cavity to affect changes in voice quality and resonance; tongue typically positioned too far back results in cul-de-sac resonance; tongue typically carried too far forward creates "thin voice" giving the baby talk effect.

- Teach clients to carry tongue in its neutral position
- Modify the excessively backward tongue position
- Modify the excessively forward tongue position
- Instruct, model, demonstrate, and reinforce correct tongue positions

Chant-Talk Method. A voice therapy technique in which words are spoken in a connected manner, with even stress, prolongation of sounds, soft glottal attack and continuously with the absence of stress for individual words; recommended for clients with hyperfunctional voice including Hard Glottal Attacks.

- Ask the patient to reduce the effort required to speak
- Play a recording of a chant and model the method

- Ask the patient to imitate the tape-recorded production by using a chant
- Ask the patient to read aloud by alternating the chant voice with the regular one
- Ask the patient to read for 20 seconds at a time
- Playback oral reading samples of the patient's voice and ask him or her to differentiate the chanted voice from the normal one
- Fade the chant and maintain normal voice without the chant

Chewing Technique. A voice therapy technique that requires patients to imagine that they are chewing food while voicing; recommended for reducing vocal hyperfunction, improving voice quality, and reducing vocal stress.

- Describe and justify the procedure to the client
- Let the client face a mirror along with you
- Ask the client to pretend that he or she is chewing some food
- Teach exaggerated open-mouth chewing motions
- Pretend to move the food from one side of the mouth to the other
- Ask the client to phonate softly various sounds by constantly moving the tongue around in chewing motions
- Ask the client to say words while chewing
- Ask the client to chew and count
- Ask the client to chew and produce connected speech
- Fade chewing movements

Digital Manipulation of the Larynx. Physical manipulation of the larynx to promote desirable voice quality; may be used to reduce vocal pitch and decrease laryngeal tension.

- Use digital pressure to lower the pitch
  - Ask the patient to prolong a vowel

  - Apply slight finger pressure to the thyroid cartilage as the vowel is prolonged (the pitch will drop)
  - Fade the digital pressure and let the client practice the lower pitch
- Lower the larynx to reduce tension
  - apply a slight downward pressure with the middle finger and the thumb just above the thyroid notch
  - ask the client to prolong vowels with larynx in the lowered position
  - use other voice facilitating techniques
  - fade the downward pressure on the larynx

Half-Swallow Boom. A method of treating low loudness and air wastage from the vocal cords; recommended for clients with Unilateral Vocal Fold Paralysis or Mutational Falsetto.

- Ask the client to swallow and as this action is still in progress, say "boom"
- Let the client produce "boom" in a low-pitched voice
- Ask the client to say "boom" louder and with less breathiness
- Have the client discriminate the normal production from the '"boom" production with the help of tape-recorded samples
- Teach the client to turn the head first to one side and then to the other and say "boom" each time
- Lower the chin while saying "boom"
- Ask the client to add sounds and words to "boom" (e.g., "boom/i/"; "boom one")
- Teach the client to add phrases and sentences
- Fade out the boom and swallow
- Ask the client to lift the chin up and bring the head back to the midline as he or she produces normal speech

Head Positioning. Manipulation of head positions to promote better voice quality; recommended especially for clients with neurological disorders including dysarthria; may be used with clients who have hyper-functional voice.

- Give instructions, model different head positions, demonstrate their effects on voice, and justify the procedure to the client
- Experiment with different head positions to find the one that promotes better voice (e.g., head rotated toward left or right; neck flexed downward with the face looking down)
- Ask the client to prolong vowels as the new head position is assumed
- Ask the client to produce longer utterances
- Gradually fade the unusual head position into a more normal position

Inhalation Phonation. A technique of voice therapy designed to evoke true vocal fold vibrations in clients who are aphonic or those who exhibit ventricular phonation.

- Raise your shoulders, inhale, and phonate a high pitched hum
- Raise your shoulders, inhale, phonate the high pitched hum and lower the shoulders, exhale, and produce the same sound; repeat this
- Teach the patient to produce inhalation phonation
- Teach the client to produce inhalation and exhalation phonation with corresponding shoulder movements
- Demonstrate the movement from the high-pitched voice to the exhaled low-pitched voice
- Reinforce the client's attempts to bring the pitch down
- Fade the shoulder movements
- Have the client practice single words until a normal sounding voice is stabilized

Masking. A technique of voice therapy to treat clients with functional aphonia and those with poor voice quality because of inadequate auditory monitoring of one's own voice; masking noise introduced through headphones.

- Use a standard audiometer to introduce masking noise; do so without any explanation
- Ask the client to read orally; turn the masking on and off for brief periods
- Tape record the client's reading to document possible changes in voice quality; or the emergence of voice in the whispering aphonic patient
- Playback the tape-recorded sample to demonstrate improved voice quality or voiced productions by an aphonic client; contrast voice with and without masking
- Ask the client to match his or her improved voice or emergence of phonation without masking
- Have the client read aloud under masking, and as the voice improves or phonation emerges, abruptly end masking; repeat this process until the client can sustain the gains

Open Mouth Approach. Oral openness during speech to increase oral resonance, reduce speaking effort, induce more relaxed speech, and to promote appropriate loudness, pitch, and quality of voice.

- Give feedback on lack of mouth opening during speech; use a mirror if necessary
- Model greater and reduced oral openness; use a puppet (greater mouth opening); contrast that with the speech of a ventriloquist (minimum mouth opening)
- Ask the client to imitate the two ways of speaking that you model
- Ask the patient to tilt the head down and speak
- Teach the client to self-monitor oral openness in natural settings
- Let the client practice speech with oral openness and reinforce for doing so

Pushing Approach. A voice therapy technique to promote better approximation of vocal cords; appropriate for increasing vocal loudness.

- Instruct and demonstrate pushing
- Ask the client to push down on the arm of the chair or push up by trying to lift the chair by gripping the bottom of the seat while seated
- Ask the client to phonate and push simultaneously
- Reinforce the louder voice that typically results
- Increase the length of utterances with the louder voice
- Fade pushing

Relaxation Training. A method to teach deep muscle relaxation with or without the help of biofeedback (e.g., electromyographic feedback); recommended for clients with excessive tension, anxiety, and stress; may be appropriate for some voice clients because of their excessive muscle tension.

- Use biofeedback instruments
- If no instruments are used, give instructions to contract and relax muscles
- Teach the client to discriminate between tensed and relaxed muscles by alternately asking him or her to tense and relax selected muscles (e.g., shoulder, neck, or jaw muscles)
- Select facial, neck, and head muscles for relaxation training; ask the client to relax one set of muscles and tense them to appreciate the difference
- Manipulate head positions to induce relaxation
- Ask the client to imagine speaking situations that induce greater tension and immediately let the client relax the speech muscles
- Use relaxing head movements (positions) if necessary
- Use other appropriate voice therapy techniques in combination with relaxation
- Stabilize a relaxed speaking posture and improved voice quality

Respiration Training. Teaching clients to manage inhalation-exhalation cycles optimally for the purpose of phonation and sustained vocalization.

- Explain the relation between breathing and speaking
- Teach the client to inhale more quickly but exhale more slowly and in a controlled manner
- Ask the client to prolong vowels to teach controlled and prolonged exhalation that would better support speech; in progressive steps, teach the client to prolong a vowel for about 20 seconds
- Teach the client to inhale quickly between utterances
- Teach good posture which promotes normal airflow management

Vocal Rest. A voice therapy technique that requires little or no talking, typically for 4–7 days; vocal rest may be complete or partial.

- Instruct the client either to totally avoid or markedly reduce
  - speaking
  - shouting or screaming
  - singing or humming
  - whispering
  - coughing or throat clearing
  - laughing or crying
  - lifting or pushing heavy objects
- Have a family member monitor these activities
- Teach the client to keep a record of such activities
- Teach the client to self-monitor

Whisper-Phonation Method. A voice therapy technique that uses Prephonation Airflow to reduce Hard Glottal Attack; the client is required to whisper sustained vowel productions; gentle phonation is introduced as the vowel is being sustained.

- Ask the client to whisper monosyllabic words that have vowel initiates

- Teach the client to whisper the initial vowel very gently
- Introduce gentle phonation as the end of the vowel is prolonged
- Gradually increase the loudness of the whisper until phonation is introduced
- Teach the client to blend the whisper into a soft phonation
- Reinforce speaking in a relaxed, breathy voice

Yawn-Sigh Method. A voice therapy technique for clients with hypervocal function; uses the relaxing effects of the inspiratory yawn followed by an expiratory sigh and phonation.

- Instruct and demonstrate the relaxing effects of prolonged inspiration involved in a yawn and the relaxed phonation that results with a sigh
- Ask the client to yawn and then exhale slowly while phonating lightly
- Ask the client to say words that start with /h/ after each yawn
- Teach the client to produce a gentle, voiced sigh while exhaling
- Teach the client to produce an easy, prolonged, open-mouthed exhalation after each yawn
- Ask the client to skip the yawn and teach the client to inhale normally and exhale a prolonged sigh with the open mouth
- Ask the patient to say "hah" after beginning each sigh
- Ask the patient to say additional words all beginning with the glottal /h/
- Ask the patient to blend in an easy, relaxed, phonation during the middle of a sigh
- Fade the sigh and move on to words, phrases, and sentences

Andrews, M. L. (1995). *Manual of voice treatment: Pediatrics through geriatrics*. San Diego, CA: Singular Publishing Group.

Boone, D. R., & McFarlane, S. C. (1988). *The voice and voice therapy* (4th ed.). Englewood Cliffs, NJ: Prentice-Hall.

Prater, R. J., & Swift, R. W. (1984). *Manual of voice therapy*. Austin, TX: Pro-Ed.

Voice Prosthesis. A small (1.8 to 3.6 cm) silicone device that has a valve at the back end and an opening at the front end; inserted into the tracheoesophageal puncture; allows air into the esophagus which vibrates; the sound is shaped into speech.

Voluntary Stuttering. A treatment target in fluent stuttering approach of Van Riper; for procedures see Stuttering, Treatment; Treatment of Stuttering: Specific Techniques or Programs.

Whole Word Accuracy (WWA). A criterion measure used in multiple-phoneme approach of articulation treatment; the entire word is judged for accuracy.

Word Combinations. The same as Phrases.

ISBN 1-56593-274-9